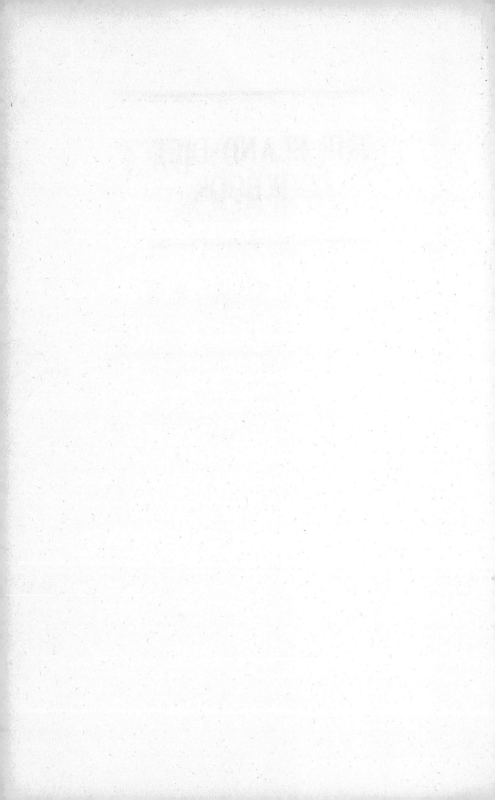

THE BLAND-DIET COOKBOOK

THE BLAND-DIET COOKBOOK

by Cecilia L. Schulz, R. N.

Introduction by
Michael R. Delman, M.D., F.A.C.G.
Assistant Clinical Professor of Medicine
SUNY, Stony Brook

G. P. Putnam's Sons · New York

TO JOHN
WITH LOVE

Contents

Author's Note

In presenting this book, I have earnestly tried to help the individual who is on a special diet which has been prescribed by a doctor. Such assistance is offered in the form of special recipes and suggested daily menus to serve as a guide to meal planning. These should make it easier for the patient to adhere to the therapeutic diet as ordered by the physician.

All but a few recipes in this book are designed to serve more than one person. In part, the reason for this is a practical one—you would find it almost impossible to prepare most dishes for the use of one person who is on a special diet unless you plan to freeze portions to be consumed by the patient on later occasions. The point to be remembered is that the recipes selected are suited not only to the patient on a bland diet. They meet his special nutritional needs, but, most important, they can be enjoyed by the entire family or by guests who, in this way, aid considerably in keeping the patient from feeling he is "odd man out." Of course, those not on a bland diet can ignore such admonitions as "do not eat the chicken skin," for example, and can use condiments with their food that must be avoided by the patient.

In no way does this volume substitute for medical care of the patient by a doctor. The reader who believes that the health information contained herein may be of personal benefit is urged to check with the physician regarding its value and also discuss any changes that may be necessitated by allergies or personal idiosyncracies.

C.L.S.

9

Acknowledgments

I wish to express grateful thanks to the many people who have helped in planning and writing this book.

To John Hargrove, my husband, whose cooperation, patience, and superior culinary prowess have been of inestimable help.

To Dr. Michael R. Delman, for his Introduction.

To Jane and Harold Grobe, for valued assistance, far over and above the call of friendship.

To the several worthy physicians, whose knowledge of nutrition, through a sympathetic professional osmosis, has taught me much, enabling me to improve my own health and to serve patients with nutritional problems more intelligently.

To Glenda Kadian, R.N., Frances Ball, R.N., Cecilia Mendl, R.N., Doris Deno, Freda Hirsch, and Felicia Setteducati, who have been most helpful in specialized fields.

To the loving relatives and cherished friends who have generously contributed recipes which, modified for use in the bland diet, form the backbone of the material in this book, along with my own collection of recipes.

C.L.S.

Introduction

by Michael R. Delman, M.D.
Fellow, American College of Gastroenterology
Assistant Clinical Professor of Medicine, SUNY, Stony Brook

Acid peptic disease, gallbladder disease, and large-bowel disease are among the most frequently encountered diseases in this country. Together, they account for untold hours of suffering and time lost from work. In 1968, Dr. Irwin S. Blumenthal, writing in the journal, *Gastroenterology*, estimated the economic loss for the United States at over one billion dollars per year for peptic ulcer alone. Although figures may vary, estimates of incidence as high as one out of every ten Americans and one out of every ten hospital admissions have been postulated for peptic ulcer.

Modern-day diets and affluence (in addition to inherited factors) have predisposed many of us to the development of acid peptic disease, gallbladder disease, and various colonic disorders. At times it is not possible or feasible to eliminate the disease process by "excision" and we must rely on alternative therapies.

Bland diets are a mainstay of treatment for many of these conditions. Low-residue and low-fat diets may also be required of the patient who already is laboring under the strain of the bland diet. The need for patient compliance cannot be sufficiently underscored and yet, when one starts hallucinating sausages, smoked fish, or pizza, the lack of compliance is readily understandable. It remained for some compassionate expert to develop a dietary schemata which would satisfy even the most epicurean of tastes. Gourmets, alas, are not immune to the development of disease.

The rapid pace of "modern" society appears to have increased the incidence of "stomach" problems. Moreover, many physicians, caught up in the time squeeze, have not been able to do much more than to hand their patients who require a bland diet a pre-printed sheet of dos and don'ts. A professional nurse has now leaped propitiously "into the breach" by compiling this comprehensive cookbook for persons ordered by their doctors on a bland diet. Cecilia L. Schulz has combined the specialized knowledge gained from long years of nursing service with her personal culinary expertise. Her volume of recipes is calculated to tantalize the taste buds of the most blasé dieter and thus to improve patient compliance.

The author is no newcomer to the world of writing. She has written several books, as well as a goodly number of articles published in nursing journals and in magazines of general interest. As a Registered Nurse, she has had opportunity to observe the reactions of patients on various therapeutic diets. To this know-how she has added her personal experiences in the kitchen and her empathy. The result was predictable—a treasury of good eating for people who, although stricken with a malady, are not willing to forgo the pleasures of the palate.

The physical suffering of a sick patient is related to the individual's mental state. With acid peptic disease, it is likely that the healing process, if not the disease process itself, is also related to the patient's emotional health. Because one of our basic drives is to eat, the withdrawal of food, even if only certain types, may produce an environment unfavorable for healing. I believe that in offering a more than satisfactory alternative, we can help speed the healing process, ease the pain of the disease, and lessen the distress of the cure.

THE BLAND-DIET COOKBOOK

1. You and Your Diet

So your doctor has recommended a therapeutic diet for you! Whatever your initial feelings may have been as you heard this medical pronouncement—shock, because you really didn't think you were that badly off; relief, because you suspected you were far worse off; annoyance, because you don't see how you can possibly interpolate a strange new set of eating rules into your present routine—you have had time, at this point, to collect your thoughts and to plan your campaign of action.

Of course, it is possible that your revised program of living has already been set out for you; that a hospital sojourn was indicated by your physician as your first step toward recovery. If so, you have become acquainted with many of the dos and don'ts connected with your rearranged "design for living." Nevertheless, the contents of these pages, covering your emotional approach to a therapeutic regime, should be as pertinent to you as are the stern and rockbound rules of diet that will govern your future eating habits.

As a nurse who has surmounted ill health by means of therapeutic diet and who has also helped a number of patients to do so, both in the home and in the hospital, I have accumulated, over the years, a wealth of classic, hand-me-down recipes. These, in modified form, together with a number of recently compiled menu creations make up the backbone of this book. Just as important, I have learned a great deal, through personal experience and observation, about the technique of living with a diet. This entails making a plan that will enable you to live securely—if not flamboyantly—through a situation that, without the correct approach, can become a horrendous ordeal and deteriorate into a miserable fiasco.

By far the most important attitude to cultivate, insofar as your

17

diet is concerned, is a cheerful acceptance. Decide from the word "go" that you will live harmoniously with the new regime, rather than exist with it resentfully, irritably, sullenly. In other words, don't fight it! Your medical checkups will reflect the constructive attitude you have assumed, just as your progress will reveal the conscientiousness with which you are abiding by your nutritional rules.

As important as your cheerful acceptance of a bad situation is your need to retain your sense of humor. There is, to be sure, nothing amusing about any form of ill health. In your particular case, the need to be reminded three or more times a day, as you sit down to your meals, that you are not precisely in the pink, does not make for riotous laughter. But if you will occasionally tell yourself how very fortunate you are, since, in the light of present-day medical knowledge, you probably can regain your health through the simple expedient of eating certain foods and not eating certain others—and, possibly, downing some oral medication—you may conclude that all is not as black as you may have thought.

Having decided that you will cheerfully accept your new diet, and that you will try to retain your sense of humor, you are ready for a third admonition. You must *determine* that your diet will succeed. Be realistic! Consider the fact that the alternatives to an unsuccessful therapeutic diet can be chronic discomfort, major surgery, or gradual deterioration of health to a more serious condition.

All too many individuals, after a valiant attempt to follow a prescribed diet, and encouraged by some amelioration of their most severe symptoms, begin to lean gradually toward the "what not to eat" side of their diet list, with foreseeable negative results. This, in medical circles, is a twice-told tale! Every experienced doctor can testify that gustatory boredom is sometimes responsible for unnecessarily prolonged illness and failure of a nutritional regime.

Even a disciplined adult, obliged to subsist, day after day, on a limited and uninteresting diet, may find it difficult to do so. Especially trying is the lot of the ambulatory patient. Able to lead an otherwise fairly normal life, exposed to the temptation of the restaurant "bill of fare" or to the invitations of friends or relatives to lunch or dine, perhaps weary of resisting the allure of the supermarket's abundant array of "no-no's," and/or frustrated by unfamiliar culinary limitations, this individual needs fortitude and will power— and several other staunch, old-fashioned qualities—if the diet is to be maintained.

The person who is determined to stick with a diet will find various methods of doing so. One way is by studying the "permitted" lists of food, provided by the doctor, and creating from them new recipes that are original and appetizing. Furthermore, by making intelligent use of the public library, the amateur cook on a restricted diet can learn from its bountiful shelves to become, if not a James Beard or a Julia Child, at least a versatile coper, capable of preparing simple, palatable meals that do not violate the therapeutic diet.

I recall a male patient, a bachelor, who, finding his therapeutic fare monotonous, developed an increasing interest in food preparation and gradually achieved extraordinarily good self-created meals. His great triumph was a dinner party to which his doctor, the girl of his dreams, and I, his erstwhile nurse, were invited, and for which he cooked and served delectable food based entirely on his diet list. Two of his original recipes are included in this book but by his request must remain anonymous.

The keynote of a successful diet is mastery of the art of compromise—learning to adjust by concession. The individual who eschews the forbidden items on the diet list and bravely substitutes items from previously unexplored, permitted areas of nutrition may happen upon a whole new world of gustatory delight.

Habitual long-term use of strong spices, alcohol, and tobacco can blunt the normal responses of the taste buds. The result of relinquishing such pleasures in the cause of improved health can be a new sensitivity to more delicate food seasonings. Gradual re-education of one's tastes can make any new diet more tolerable.

The modern bland-diet "permitted" list boasts many herbs and flavorings. Although they may be less robust, less exciting, less exotic, than those enjoyed on the average, everyday, normal diet, they can, if judiciously employed, enhance bland-diet meals and make dietary deprivations less acute.

The meal which might have seemed, in pre-bland-diet days, an array of uninteresting "blah" dishes can be transformed into a Lucullan feast if one exercises "adjustment by concession," giving up forbidden foods in order to enjoy new flavors, new methods of preparation, new tastes.

2. Cooking for the Bland-Diet Patient

No matter how many cooking courses one has benefited by, no matter how many years one has cooked, successfully, for an appreciative family, no matter how many cookbooks one has collected and enjoyed, it is essential to master the techniques of bland-diet cooking if that is to be the order of the day. Although most of the fundamental rules of cooking remain the same, a few do not. Furthermore, it is wise to acquaint oneself with the equipment used in bland-diet cookery, which can facilitate food preparation tremendously. To learn even one shortcut or one more effective method of preparing meals for the patient on a therapeutic diet is to make life easier for the patient and the cook as well.

Logically, first consideration should be given the preparation of meat, since it is one of the prime sources of *protein,* the food constituent that builds and repairs tissues. (Lest there be any question about the status of protein, one can refer to its Greek root which means "primary" or "of the first importance.")

Roasting, broiling, and panbroiling are the most frequently indicated methods of cooking meat on the bland diet. Frying is out of the picture entirely. Fat and gristle are removed whenever possible before cooking.

Roasting. When cooking a roast, place it on the rack that comes with your roasting pan. This prevents it from stewing in its own juice.

There are two classic methods of cooking a roast. One calls for searing it first—placing it briefly in a very hot oven, then, after a short period, lowering the heat to moderate temperature which will be retained for the remainder of the roasting time. This results in a crisp crust with a juicy interior. The second method consists of

21

cooking the roast at a constant, low temperature throughout the entire cooking period. This yields a less crisp crust, but the interior is juicier and generally more tender.

Broiling is an excellent way to cook steaks and chops quickly. A simple and practical method of broiling involves preheating the oven to 500 degrees, lightly oiling the broiler pan, and placing the meat on it, about three or four inches from the source of heat. When the steak or chop is seared on the top side, it is turned and seared on the other side. Broiling is continued until the desired degree of doneness is reached. Total broiling time is, of course, dependent on the thickness of the meat.

Panbroiling—cooking on top of the stove in a Dutch oven or heavy skillet—may be done without the use of any oil or fat by simply sprinkling some salt in the very hot pan before placing steaks or chops in it for cooking. Meat patties—hamburgers—can be cooked this way as well. Or one can use the no-fat, no-calorie, no-taste vegetable spray made to coat cookware.

For cooking chicken, each recipe usually explains the cooking procedure. In bland-food preparation frying is contraindicated. Chicken and other poultry may be roasted, broiled, poached, simmered, baked in casseroles or soufflés, or roto-broiled on a spit.

Variety Meats (Organ Meats and Glands)—sweetbreads, fresh tongue (smoked tongue and all other smoked foods are on the "no-no" list), heart, brains, kidneys, and liver—which possess high nutritive value and whose texture makes them especially suitable for a bland diet, may be cooked in various ways. Liver—whether steer, calf, or chicken—is usually panbroiled, sometimes baked, or made into a loaf. Sweetbreads and brains are simmered and served in a cream sauce; kidneys may be sautéed, baked, or broiled; fresh tongue is simmered and served with a sauce; beef heart may be stewed or combined with other ingredients into a meat loaf. Since some persons may not have been gastronomically educated to enjoy organ meats and glands, which are regarded as special delicacies by others, the cook may choose—after wrestling with his or her conscience—to disguise them in the cooking and serve them under an assumed name.

Fish rates a place of honor on the bland-diet list. It has many virtues—it is an excellent source of protein, contains an abundance of vitamins and minerals, and is comparatively low in calories. Smoked and salted fish are not on the bland-diet "approved" list—but fresh, frozen, and some canned fish serve in numerous versatile rôles.

Fish may be cooked in many ways: broiled, baked, pan-broiled, poached, and steamed. Whichever method you choose, an important precaution should be observed—do not overcook fish!

Broiling is an easy way to cook fish. Split small whole fish down the back, or use fillets. Sprinkle the fish lightly with salt and lemon juice. Place a whole fish, skin-side down, on a greased broiler and broil for ten minutes, or until the fish is nicely browned. Turn and broil it on the other side, letting the skin get brown. To broil fish fillets, brush them with melted margarine and brown them equally on both sides. (Use a pancake turner to turn the fillets.) Serve them with melted margarine, a wedge of lemon, and a sprinkle of chopped parsley or paprika.

Baking is another simple way to cook fish fillets or steaks. After drizzling a bit of melted margarine over the fish, and sprinkling lightly with salt, place it in a moderately hot oven and bake it, uncovered, for twenty-five minutes or so, or until it flakes readily. Serve the fish on a hot plate, garnished with finely chopped parsley, and a lemon wedge.

Fish that is to be poached—usually a large fish or thick slices of fish—is wrapped in cheesecloth, placed in a kettle and covered with hot (not boiling) water, to which has been added one-half teaspoon salt and one-half-tablespoon lemon juice for each quart used. Bring the water to the boiling point and let the fish simmer, covered, until it separates from the bone. Drain and serve it on a hot platter with an egg sauce (page 125).

Cooked or canned fish lends itself to many intriguing main dishes. It may be served with a simple sauce, mixed with mashed potatoes, incorporated into a soufflé, creamed and served in a noodle ring, or used in a casserole, a fish loaf, or a mousse.

There are many fancy, even ambrosial methods of preparing fish—with wine, with delectable, fussy sauces, with exotic garnishing—but they are not for the bland-diet patient. However, a four-star rating is earned by simply cooked fish, appetizingly presented as part of a well-balanced meal.

Shellfish. If you ask an aficionado, shellfish provide more palate-pleasure per calorie than any other kind of food. Of infinite variety, these fruits of the sea lend themselves to many different kinds of preparation. Insofar as the bland diet is concerned, it is necessary to check with one's personal physician when it comes to enjoying shellfish. Oysters and clams may be permitted, but controversy may exist over scallops, mussels, snails, lobsters, crabs, and shrimp.

Oysters make versatile bland-diet fare, except in recipes that call for frying, strong spices, rich sauces, or the use of wine. Whether served as appetizers, soups, chowders, bisques, or mid-meal snacks—whether boiled, broiled, baked, scalloped, creamed, or in a casserole—they are invariably listed in the "treat" category. While it must be admitted that oysters are not in the economy class, an occasional splurge might be regarded as a reward of merit for the patient who has adhered to some of the more spartan aspects of the bland diet.

Vegetables and Fruits. One of the most elementary—but efficient—ways to cook fruits and vegetables is to steam them. Flavor is retained by placing the particular food in a covered strainer over boiling water until it is cooked. In this way precious vitamins are not lost in discarded cooking water.

A recently developed type of vegetable steamer is made of stainless steel, has self-adjusting sides that fit most pots, and folds compactly for easy storage. In addition to being a highly practical item, it is also most attractive in appearance and can be used as a serving dish as well as a steamer.

Fruits and vegetables can be boiled without a major loss of food constituents if very little water is used and if the cook stands by to make sure that the pot doesn't boil dry, thus scorching the contents.

Strained and mashed fruits and vegetables are called for in a number of recipes planned for the early convalescent stage of the bland diet for peptic ulcer. Straining fruits and vegetables after they are cooked isn't all that difficult. If you use a blender, make sure to follow the manufacturer's instructions carefully. You can also use a wire strainer or a metal colander, with an old-fashioned wooden potato masher, or a pastry blender, or a newer type of metal masher. Or you can use a food mill, in which a rotating handle attached to a flat plate pushes the pulp of the fruit or vegetable through holes in the bottom.

It's important to remember that peels, seeds, and tough fibers do not a bland diet make. Avoid all roughage!

Baby foods are helpful in preparing some bland-diet dishes, especially those used in the early convalescent stage of the peptic-ulcer diet. The producers who specialize in baby foods—which include meat as well as fruits and vegetables—can provide some excellent recipes for the asking.

The pressure cooker may be used in preparing various foods—meat, fish, vegetables, cereals, soups, et cetera—for the bland diet. Its virtues include economy of cooking fuel and time, but, most important, food flavors, vitamins, and minerals are preserved. In ordinary cooking methods, much of the vitamin content of foods, particularly Vitamin C, may be lost through oxidation and prolonged cooking. In the pressure cooker, foods are cooked in the shortest possible time. If you use the pressure cooker, you must learn how to handle it. A booklet usually accompanies the cooker and it is a wise precaution to study it assiduously.

Salads. The bland-diet salad presents a real challenge to the cook, since it lacks all the qualifications usually identified with a good salad. It is definitely *not* composed of crisp, raw greens, fresh raw vegetables, fresh raw fruits, pungent herbs, exciting spices, delectable garnishing, piquant dressing.

However, by using the ingredients permitted, in the manner suggested, the cook can concoct salads that feature color, variety, and taste. Because their vitamin and mineral content make them valuable adjuncts to bland-diet fare, they should be incorporated frequently into the menu.

Among the salad recipes for the bland diet, molded salads with a gelatin base have eye-and-taste appeal. As the patient progresses from the early convalescent stage of strained or mashed ingredients, his salads may contain soft canned or frozen fruits and vegetables, cream or cottage cheese, and yogurt (except on the low-fat diet or the low-residue diet where the physician has restricted the consumption of dairy products).

Desserts on the bland diet cover a wide range of good things to eat. Important among them are cooked and strained fruits. Fruit desserts during early convalescence can be made of the puréed baby foods mentioned earlier. These are especially helpful if you live alone and prepare your own meals.

Gelatins provide variety and interest. They may consist of the unflavored, colorless kind which you yourself transform into a finished product, employing the cooked fruits, vegetables, and juices on your list, or they may be the already flavored gelatins which require little time and effort to convert into shimmering, appetizing, easily digested additions to your meals.

Custards and old-fashioned puddings may also be eaten as desserts, although these substantial dishes should be taken after a light lunch or supper. There is also a large variety of pleasant, nourishing, easily prepared or already prepared desserts, such as junket rennet, yogurt, and fruited-cottage-cheese dishes (except on the low-fat diet or the low-residue diet where dairy products have been limited).

Ice cream has a special value insofar as palate-pleasure and nourishment are concerned, but it cannot be consumed on the low-fat diet. Then there are less-robust desserts such as sherbets and ice milk, which should not be overlooked, unless the patient must avoid dairy products as in the low-fat diet.

An important fact to be remembered—especially if you have the proverbial "sweet tooth" and are preparing or ordering your own meals—is keep your menu balanced. At luncheon, don't skip blithely from a cream-cheese-and-jelly sandwich to a rich pudding slathered with whipped cream. At dinner, remember the value of protein, in the form of meat, fish, or an occasional egg dish, and the four-star importance of vegetables and fruits. Let the dessert be *la bonne bouche* of the repast—but only that—not the "special feature attraction"!

3. The Bland Diet for Peptic Ulcer

The bland diet is composed of foods intended to soothe; that is, foods which are smooth in texture and mild in flavor. The following pages include an outline of the type of diet which the doctor may order for peptic ulcer. This diet may also be prescribed by the physician for chronic indigestion, "dyspepsia," or "squeamish" stomach. For a hiatus-hernia patient, especially one who is overweight, the doctor may order a bland diet with lowered calories in order to prevent superfluous tissue from pressing against the diaphragm.

For many years, a treatment frequently ordered for the hospitalized ulcer patient was the one named for the doctor who first proposed it in 1915—Dr. Bertram Welton Sippy. The Sippy diet consisted of feedings of half cream and half milk, administered every hour until the patient went to sleep for the night. The theory behind this treatment was to counteract the acidity of the stomach by constantly coating it with soothing, soft food. Medication and rest were included in the routine ulcer treatment, along with the Sippy diet. The milk-cream diet was gradually augmented with a bland cooked cereal, such as Cream of Wheat, served with milk. Soft-boiled eggs and cream soups rounded out the early stage of the regime.

The Sippy diet is now somewhat modified in certain hospitals, but an integral phase of the ulcer patient's treatment still hinges on a soothing, nonirritating diet, combined with rest and proper medication.

During early convalescence, the patient's food may consist of fluids, semi-solids, strained and soft nourishment. Chopped meat is usually ordered when the ulcer patient has passed the initial stage of convalescence. The physician specifies precisely when meat is to be added to the diet, and also the amount which is to be served at any meal. The physician's "go ahead" is also given at the stage of recovery when meat, vegetables, and fruits need no longer be chopped, mashed, puréed, or strained.

Meal-spacing is an outstanding characteristic of the ulcer regimen. In addition to three meals a day, the ulcer patient's schedule includes between-meal and bedtime nourishment.

Permitted and Forbidden Foods

(To be checked, changed, augmented, by the physician according to the patient's personal need.)

PERMITTED

AVOID

BEVERAGES

Milk—whole, skimmed, modified skimmed, evaporated skimmed, buttermilk, dried non-fat milk powder. Cream, plain or diluted with milk. Yogurt.

Coffee or tea (except with the doctor's permission). Alcoholic and carbonated beverages.

SOUPS

Cream soups during early convalescence—Cream Sauce or Thin White Sauce blended with asparagus tips, peas, green beans, spinach, potatoes, carrots, tomatoes, using mashed, puréed, or strained cooked vegetables, which may be fresh, frozen, or canned. Puréed baby-food vegetables may be used.

As the patient progresses—soups may be made of all *permitted* vegetables.

Soups made with meat or meat stocks. Very hot or very cold soups.

PERMITTED	**AVOID**

VEGETABLES

During early convalescence—fresh, frozen, canned—cooked puréed, strained, or mashed asparagus tips, peas, green beans, spinach, potatoes, tomatoes, carrots. *As the patient progresses*—tender beets, mushrooms, acorn and summer squash, sweet and white potatoes, yams, cream-style canned corn. All must be cooked until tender, but, with the doctor's permission, they need no longer be strained. Raw lettuce, finely shredded, and diced tomatoes, skin and seeds removed, but only with the doctor's permission.	Strong-flavored vegetables—onions, cabbage, cauliflower, Brussels sprouts, radishes, cucumbers, turnips. Seeds, skins, or rough fibers of any vegetable. Raw vegetables except raw lettuce if the doctor approves its use.

FRUITS

Fruit juices during early convalescence—orange and grapefruit juice, strained, diluted with water, served at the end of breakfast. *Fruit juices as the patient progresses*—prune (strained), apple, cranberry; apricot, pear, and peach nectar. *Fruits during convalescence*—strained, mashed, or puréed (baby-food fruits may be used) apples, apricots, cherries, berries, peaches, pears, bananas. Fruits may be fresh, canned, or frozen, but fresh and frozen fruits must be cooked and all must be strained. *Fruits as the patient progresses*—the same cooked fruits as in early convalescence, but the doctor may give permission to serve well-cooked fruits without straining. Raw bananas and avocados.	Raw fruits, except bananas and avocados.

PERMITTED	AVOID

MEAT

Meat during early convalescence— Ground lean beef patties, broiled or panbroiled. Meat loaf.
*As the patient progresses—*beef, lamb, veal (tender cuts, cooked thoroughly). Poultry of all kinds. Organ meats.

Meat fat or gristle. Pork. Smoked or preserved meat. Cold cuts. Fried meat.

FISH

*As the patient progresses—*fish fillets and fish steaks (poached, broiled, or baked). Fish timbales, soufflés, casseroles (with permitted ingredients). Water-packed canned tuna or salmon (with the doctor's permission).

Fried fish. Raw fish. Smoked, highly seasoned fish. Fatty fish, such as mackerel, bluefish, lake trout, butterfish.

FATS

Margarine, butter, cream, vegetable fats, oils.

Commercial salad dressings. Mineral oil. Excessive use of fats. Fried foods.

EGGS

Number per week, according to doctor's order. Cooked in any way except fried.

Fried eggs.

CHEESE

Cottage and cream cheese. Mild American cheese for cooking.

Strong, sharp, spicy cheeses.

30

PERMITTED	AVOID

BREADS, CEREALS, PASTAS

Plain rolls, enriched white bread, soda crackers, rusk, zwieback, rye bread without seeds, hard rolls. Strained oatmeal, cream of wheat, farina, rice (white). Macaroni, noodles, and spaghetti.	Sweet rolls, pretzels, seeded rolls, salty crackers, whole-wheat bread, graham bread, other coarse breads. Brown rice and wild rice.

DESSERTS

Fruits—canned, fresh, frozen (the last two must be cooked). Gelatin—plain or with allowed fruits. Puddings—rice, bread, tapioca, cornstarch. Custard, junket, ice cream, sherbet, ice milk. Cakes and cookies, simple, not rich or overly sweet.	Nuts and seeds. Excessively sweet or rich desserts.

SEASONINGS

Allspice, cinnamon, mace, lemon, paprika, parsley, sage, salt, and thyme (in moderation).	Garlic, pepper, and onion.

As the Patient Progresses

When the physician sees fit, the patient on the bland diet for peptic ulcer is promoted from early convalescent foods to a more advanced regime. The food restrictions on the original "not permitted" list remain valid as the patient's health improves, but whether or not meats, vegetables, and fruits should still be puréed, strained, or mashed is a question for the doctor to decide. A number of recipes in this section include chopped ingredients. These, however, will be found in dishes somewhat more sophisticated than those of the simple early convalescent diet.

In addition, following the early stage of convalescence, persons on the bland diet for peptic ulcer may use the recipes designed for the bland low-residue diet and the bland low-fat diet, with the exception of recipes for soups containing a meat base, stews, and gravies.

Discreet use of the various delicate seasonings permitted as the patient progresses can help to make meals more palatable and more intriguing.

The manner in which the recuperating patient consumes food is of great importance. A relaxed mealtime mood is not always easily achieved if one is tense by nature and/or harassed by worrisome problems, but a peaceful state of mind should be a major objective in the process of attaining permanent good health. Today many constructive means exist by which the average individual, under stress, can learn to overcome, or at least to deal with, tension.

Certainly, attention should be given to the simple, specific rules of mealtime hygiene. The patient should eat slowly, chew thoroughly, restrict fluid to one glass per meal, and sip it slowly. Other considerations include a pleasant, leisurely, relaxed atmosphere, varied menus, and attractively served meals. Extremely hot or cold dishes should be avoided.

Soups (Early Convalescence)

Soups for the patient with peptic ulcer are divided into two categories. The first is most helpful during early convalescence.

Fresh, frozen, or canned vegetables may be used for these soups. Fresh vegetables should be boiled, covered, in a small amount of water, or steamed over boiling water. Frozen vegetables are to be cooked according to the directions on the package. Canned vegetables need no further cooking. Whether fresh, frozen, or canned, all vegetables during early convalescence must be strained or puréed. Puréed baby foods are often used in the preparation of cream of vegetable soups in early convalescence.

The Thin White Sauce (page 123) is most useful in making cream of vegetable soups. Half a cup of strained vegetable added to one cup of the white sauce, smoothly blended, and simmered for five minutes over low heat, or heated in the top of a double boiler, makes two small servings.

Cream of Asparagus Soup

½ cup canned asparagus
   tips

1 cup Thin White Sauce
   (page 123)

Pour the asparagus tips into a strainer, draining the liquid from the can into a bowl. Mash the asparagus tips, using a potato masher or a pastry blender, or push them through the strainer. Combine the asparagus with the reserved liquid. Prepare the sauce in a medium saucepan. Add the strained asparagus tips and the liquid to the sauce. Mix thoroughly. Simmer, stirring frequently. The soup should be served warm, not hot.

Yield: 2 servings

Cream of Green Bean Soup

2 cups Thin White Sauce
   (page 123)

1 cup canned green beans,
   drained
   Salt

Prepare the sauce in a four-cup saucepan. Set aside. Purée the beans in the blender and add them to the sauce. Mix thoroughly. Add salt to taste. Simmer over low heat, stirring constantly. The soup should be served warm, not hot.

Yield: 4 servings

Cream of Green Pea Soup

1 cup Thin White Sauce
   (page 123)

½ cup canned green peas

Prepare the sauce in a medium saucepan. In a separate saucepan, heat the peas in the liquid from the can for ten minutes. Drain the peas. Force them through a sieve or a food mill. Add them to the sauce. Mix the two ingredients thoroughly. Simmer for ten minutes. Beat the soup vigorously with a whisk or rotary beater before serving. It should be served warm, not hot.

Yield: 2 servings

Cream of Potato Soup

3 small potatoes	1 egg, slightly beaten
2 cups Thin White Sauce (page 123)	⅛ teaspoon salt

Peel and cube the potatoes. Place them in a medium saucepan in just enough water to cover, and cook, tightly covered, for about fifteen minutes, or until they are soft. While the potatoes are cooking, prepare the sauce in the top of a double boiler. Mash the potatoes. Add the egg and the salt. Mix thoroughly with the sauce. Cool the soup somewhat before serving.

Yield: 4 servings

Cream of Carrot Soup

1 cup Thin White Sauce (page 123)	1 large carrot

Prepare the sauce in a medium pan. Set aside. Scrape the carrot and slice it thickly. Place the slices in a regular steamer or in a suitable strainer. Cover, and steam over a saucepan containing boiling water. When the carrot slices test fork-tender, remove them from the steamer and push them through a sieve or food mill. Add the carrot pulp to the sauce. Simmer, stirring constantly, until well mixed, about ten minutes. Cool slightly before serving.

Yield: 2 servings

Cream of Spinach Soup

1   cup chopped frozen
    spinach
	2 cups Thin White Sauce
	    (page 123)
	4 tablespoons sour cream

Prepare the frozen spinach according to the directions on the package. Push the cooked spinach through a sieve, or purée in a blender, using the amount of liquid indicated in the manufacturer's instruction manual. Prepare the sauce. Combine the spinach with the sauce in the top of a double boiler or in a medium saucepan. Heat thoroughly. Serve warm, not hot, with a dollop of sour cream.

Yield: 4 servings

Cream of Tomato Soup

1	one-pound twelve-ounce can tomatoes	2	tablespoons flour
1	teaspoon sugar	2	tablespoons margarine
1	teaspoon salt	1¾	cups milk

Combine the first three ingredients in a two-quart saucepan. Simmer for ten minutes. Sieve to remove seeds. Prepare the Thin White Sauce (page 123), using the flour, margarine, and milk but omitting the salt specified in the standard recipe. Slowly add the hot tomato mixture to the sauce, stirring constantly. Cool slightly before serving.

Yield: 5 servings

Soups (As the Patient Progresses)

Note: The following recipes are to be used, with the doctor's permission, after the early stage of convalescence.

Cream of Beet Soup

2	cups Thin White Sauce (page 123)	1	cup strained beets (baby food may be used)
		3	tablespoons sour cream

Prepare the sauce in a medium saucepan. Add the beets to the sauce. Mix thoroughly. Simmer for about five minutes. Serve in mugs. Top with a dollop of sour cream.

Yield: 3 servings

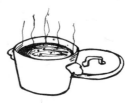

Borsch, American Style

2	cups canned sliced beets	3	cups water
¾	cup beet juice	1	sprig parsley, chopped very fine
2	tablespoons sugar		
¼	teaspoon salt		Thyme
2	tablespoons lemon juice	½	cup sour cream, whipped

Purée the beets in the blender, using the amount of fluid required according to the manufacturer's instruction manual. Or chop the beets finely and push through a food mill. In a medium saucepan combine the beets, beet juice, sugar, salt, lemon juice, water, parsley, and a sprinkle of thyme. Bring to a boil. Simmer for about eight minutes. Remove from the heat and chill. Serve cold, but not icy. Top with the sour cream.

Yield: 5 servings

Cream of Corn Soup

2½	cups cream-style canned corn, strained	2	egg yolks
2	cups Thin White Sauce (page 123)	1	cup evaporated milk
			Paprika
			Soda crackers (optional)

Combine the puréed corn with the sauce in the top of a double boiler. Heat. Beat the egg yolks. Add the evaporated milk gradually to the egg yolks. Whisk into the soup. Heat. Pour into five mugs. Sprinkle lightly with paprika. Soda crackers may be crumbled into the individual servings.

Yield: 5 servings

Cream of Green Bean Soup with Cheese

2	cups finely cut fresh green beans	3	cups Thin White Sauce (page 123)
1	tablespoon finely minced parsley	¼	cup grated mild American cheese
½	teaspoon salt		Paprika

Add the beans and the parsley to enough salted boiling water to cover in a medium saucepan. Simmer, covered, for twenty minutes or until the beans are soft. Strain. Prepare the sauce. Add the beans and the parsley to the sauce. Stir, blending thoroughly. Heat. Serve in soup plates. Sprinkle the cheese over each serving. Top with a dash of paprika.

Yield: 6 servings

Cream of Mushroom Soup

1½ cups mushrooms	3 cups Thin White Sauce
Mace	(page 123)
	Salt

Cut the mushrooms into very small pieces. Simmer, with a dash of mace, in just enough water to cover, for five minutes. Add to the sauce. Heat for five minutes. Salt lightly.

Yield: 6 servings

Cream of Mushroom and Spinach Soup

Cream of Mushroom	above)
Soup—six servings (see	2 cups raw spinach

Prepare the mushroom soup according to the recipe. Wash the spinach thoroughly. Chop very fine. Add the spinach to the soup. Mix well. Simmer gently for five minutes.

Yield: 6 servings

Oyster Soup Special

1 pint oysters	1 cup milk
3 cups hot water	1 egg yolk, lightly beaten
1 sprig parsley, finely chopped	½ cup light cream (or evaporated milk)
Salt	Mace

Pick over the oysters. Remove any bits of shell. Heat in their own liquor until the edges curl. Strain, reserving the liquor. Chop

37

the oysters. Bring the oyster liquor, water, parsley, and salt (to taste) to a boil in a medium saucepan. Combine the milk, egg yolk, and cream and add to the saucepan. Simmer gently for three minutes, stirring constantly. Add the chopped oysters. Heat thoroughly. Serve warm with a light dusting of mace.

Yield: 5 to 6 servings

Oyster Stew

1 pint oysters	1 quart milk
4 tablespoons margarine	Paprika
Salt	Oysterette crackers

Pick over the oysters, removing any bits of shell. Strain the oyster liquor. Place the oysters, oyster liquor, margarine, and salt to taste in a medium saucepan. Simmer gently until the oysters begin to curl at the edges. Heat the milk. Add the hot milk to the oysters. Dust lightly with paprika. Serve at once. Oysterette crackers go well with the stew.

Yield: 5 servings

Tomato Consomme, Jelled

1 envelope unflavored gelatin	1½ cups tomato juice
2 tablespoons cold water	2 tablespoons sour cream
	4 soda crackers

Soften the gelatin in the cold water. Heat the tomato juice to the boiling point. Combine the hot juice with the gelatin, stirring the mixture until the gelatin is entirely dissolved. Pour into two bouillon cups, or two small bowls. When the soup has cooled, put it into the refrigerator to set. Serve the jelled consommé with a topping of sour cream and with crackers on the side.

Yield: 2 servings

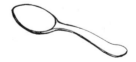

Vegetable Chowder

3 cups Thin White Sauce (page 123)	½ cup cream-style canned corn
½ cup finely chopped canned green beans	1 tablespoon finely chopped parsley
½ cup sliced canned mushrooms	1 teaspoon allspice

Prepare the sauce. Add the remaining ingredients. Blend well. Heat and serve.

Yield: 6 servings

Meat (Early Convalescence)

In ordering meat for the ulcer patient who has achieved some degree of convalescence, the doctor usually specifies that it be ground. The amount of meat to be served at each meal, and the particular day on which it is to be added to the patient's diet, is strictly the physician's jurisdiction.

It is wise to select a lean piece of meat and have it freshly ground rather than buy packaged ground meat which may be richly studded with particles of fat.

The repertory of ground-meat cookery is not extensive for those on a bland diet for peptic ulcer. However, the cook with imagination can conjure up many different ways of preparing the patient's meat dishes during early convalescence so that they add pleasure and interest to each day's menu. Frying is taboo. Broiling, pan-broiling, and baking—in the form of meat loaves or casseroles, soufflés or timbales—are cooking techniques that offer challenge and excellent results.

Applesauce Meat Loaf

1 pound lean ground beef
1 cup soft white bread crumbs
1 cup applesauce
1 egg, beaten

1 tablespoon light brown sugar
½ teaspoon salt
¼ teaspoon cinnamon

Combine all the ingredients. Mix well. Form into a loaf. Bake in a greased medium loaf pan at 350 degrees for one hour.
Yield: 4 to 6 servings

Broiled Ground Beef

1 pound lean ground beef
1 teaspoon salt

1 tablespoon margarine, melted

Shape the meat into four patties, each three-quarters of an inch thick, mixing the salt into them in the process. Brush on both sides, sparingly, with the margarine. Broil three inches away from the source of heat. After five to eight minutes, turn the patties, using a pancake turner. Broil the other side for four minutes.
Yield: servings for the patient dependent on the doctor's order

Company Beef Loaf

1½ pounds lean ground beef
1 cup white bread crumbs made from day-old bread
2 eggs, beaten
1 cup canned tomatoes, strained

1 tablespoon finely chopped parsley
Dash of thyme
Dash of sage
¼ teaspoon salt
Special Tomato Sauce (page 126)

Combine all the ingredients except the sauce. Mix thoroughly. Shape into a round loaf. Bake in a greased medium casserole at 350 degrees for one hour and fifteen minutes. Serve with the sauce.
Yield: 6 to 8 servings

Fruity Meat Loaf

1 pound lean ground beef	halves, drained
¾ cup zwieback crumbs	3 tablespoons light brown
½ teaspoon salt	sugar
1 egg, well beaten	¼ teaspoon cinnamon
¾ cup milk	1 tablespoon margarine,
2 cups canned apricot	melted

Combine the first five ingredients. Set aside. Arrange the apricot halves in the bottom of a greased medium casserole. (If desired, reserve the drained liquid for future use in a beverage.) Combine the sugar, cinnamon, and margarine. Pour over the apricots. Top with the meat mixture. Bake at 350 degrees for one hour.

Yield: 4 to 5 servings

Half-and-Half Meat Loaf

½ pound lean ground beef	1½ cups zwieback crumbs
½ pound lean ground lamb	2 sprigs parsley, finely
1 egg	chopped
1 teaspoon salt	½ teaspoon allspice
1 cup milk	

Combine all the ingredients. Mix well. Form into a medium loaf. Bake in a well-greased medium loaf pan at 350 degrees for one hour.

Yield: 6 servings

Panbroiled Ground Beef

1 pound lean ground beef	1 teaspoon salt

Form the meat into four or five smooth, round patties about one-half-inch thick. Preheat an ungreased iron skillet until it is sizzling hot. Sprinkle the salt in a thin layer over the bottom of the skillet. Cook the patties quickly over high heat. When brown, turn with a pancake turner. Brown the other side. Turn off the heat. Cover the skillet. After about five minutes, check the patties for interior doneness. They should be tender, juicy, and medium-rare.

Yield: servings for the patient dependent on the doctor's order

Sour Cream Meat Loaf

1½	slices dry white bread crumbs	¼	teaspoon salt
¾	cup sour cream	1	egg, beaten
1	pound lean ground beef	¼	teaspoon mace
			Paprika

Soften the crumbs in the sour cream. Combine with the meat, salt, egg, and mace. Mix thoroughly. Form into a loaf. Bake in a well-greased medium loaf pan at 350 degrees for one hour and twenty minutes. Dust lightly with paprika before serving.

Yield: 4 to 6 servings

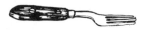

Tomato-Rice Meat Loaf

1	pound lean ground beef	¼	teaspoon salt
1	cup tomato juice	2	sprigs parsley, finely chopped
1	cup cooked white rice		
2	eggs, beaten	½	teaspoon allspice

Combine all the ingredients. Mix well. Form into a round loaf. Bake in a well-greased medium casserole at 350 degrees for one hour.

Yield: 4 to 6 servings

Carrot Beef Loaf

2	medium carrots, scraped		crumbs
1	four-ounce can mushrooms, drained	1	cup tomato juice
		1	egg, beaten
1	pound lean ground beef	½	teaspoon allspice
1	cup soft white bread		

Grate the carrots. Combine with the remaining ingredients. Bake in a well-greased medium baking pan at 350 degrees for one hour.

Yield: 4 to 6 servings

Meat (As the Patient Progresses)

Baked Chicken Breasts

1 lemon, cut in half	1 teaspoon salt
2 whole chicken breasts, split	1 tablespoon finely chopped parsley
2 tablespoons margarine, melted	½ cup pineapple juice
	¼ teaspoon allspice

Drizzle lemon juice over the chicken breasts four hours before mealtime. Refrigerate for two hours. Bring the chicken to room temperature. Preheat the oven to 350 degrees. Combine the remaining ingredients in a small bowl. Brush the mixture over the entire surface of the chicken. Place chicken, skin side up, in a shallow baking pan. Cover with aluminum foil. Bake for forty minutes. Uncover. Bake fifteen to twenty minutes longer or until the chicken breasts are fork-tender. (The patient should not eat the chicken skin.)

Yield: 4 servings

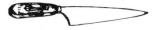

Broiled Beef Liver

1 pound beef liver (cut into slices one-half-inch thick)	2 tablespoons margarine, melted
	Salt
	Paprika

43

Cut off any membrane edging the liver. Snip out any veins with a scissors. Dip the liver slices in the margarine. Preheat the broiler. Grease the broiler pan. Broil the liver three inches away from the source of heat for three minutes. Turn and salt lightly. Broil three minutes longer. Sprinkle lightly with paprika.

Yield: 4 servings

Broiled Lamb Chops

2 loin, rib, or shoulder chops	Lemon-Margarine Sauce (page 125)
Salt	

Preheat the broiler five to ten minutes. Remove excess fat from the chops. Place them on a greased rack in the broiling pan. Broil about two inches away from the source of heat. When brown, turn, using tongs or a pancake turner, to avoid piercing the meat. Salt the second side and brown. Allow ten to fifteen minutes for chops that are three-quarters to one inch thick; eighteen to twenty-five minutes if one and one-half inches thick; twenty-eight to thirty-five minutes if two inches thick. Serve with the sauce.

Yield: 2 servings

Broiled Sweetbreads

3 pairs sweetbreads	Lemon-Margarine Sauce (page 125)
Lemon juice	
Salt	

Wash the sweetbreads immediately after buying them and put them in cold water for one hour. Drain. Place them in boiling water. Add one tablespoon of lemon juice and one teaspoon of salt to each quart of water. Simmer the sweetbreads, covered, for twenty minutes. Drain. Cover with cold water to whiten them and keep their flesh firm. When the sweetbreads are cool enough to handle, remove the membrane and the tubes. To broil, split the sweetbreads crosswise. Sprinkle lightly with salt. Preheat broiler and broil three inches away from the source of heat for about ten minutes. Turn them so both sides are browned. Serve with the sauce.

Yield: 3 to 6 servings, depending on the doctor's order

Sutton Place Sweetbreads

3 pairs sweetbreads
Salt
Lemon juice
1 ten-ounce package
frozen green peas

2 cups Medium White
Sauce (page 124)
3 cups mashed potatoes
Mace

Immediately after buying the sweetbreads, wash and place them in cold water to cover for one hour. Drain. Cover with boiling water to which 1 teaspoon of salt and 1 tablespoon of lemon juice have been added for each quart of water. Simmer, covered, for twenty minutes. Drain. Cool. When cool enough to handle, remove the membrane and the tubes. Cut into serving-size pieces. Set aside. Cook the green peas according to the package directions. Drain. Prepare the sauce. Combine the cut-up sweetbreads with the peas. Add to the sauce. Blend thoroughly. Heat. Serve over the hot mashed potatoes. Sprinkle lightly with mace.

Yield: 3 to 6 servings, depending on the doctor's order

Sweetbreads and Mushrooms

1 cup cut-up cooked
sweetbreads (see
preceding recipe)
1 cup Parsley Sauce (page
125)
1 teaspoon lemon juice

1 four-ounce can
mushrooms, drained
4 slices day-old white
bread, toasted
Paprika

Be sure to cook the sweetbreads the day you buy them. Prepare the sauce in the top of a double boiler. Add the lemon juice. Blend in the sweetbreads and mushrooms. Serve on toast. Sprinkle lightly with paprika.

Yield: 4 servings

Sweetbreads and Oyster Luncheon Treat

2 cups Medium White
Sauce (page 124)
4 pairs sweetbreads

1 pint oysters
¼ teaspoon mace
2 cups cooked white rice

Prepare the sauce in a large saucepan. Prepare the sweetbreads according to the Sutton Place Sweetbreads recipe (p. 45). Add to the sauce. Blend well. Pick over the oysters. Remove any bits of shell. Add the oysters and their liquor to the sweetbreads and the sauce. Mix thoroughly. Simmer gently, stirring occasionally, for twenty minutes. Sprinkle lightly with mace. Serve on the hot rice.

Yield: 4 to 8 servings

Lamb en Brochette

1½	pounds lamb, cut into one-inch squares	½	cup melted margarine
6	slices canned pineapple, cut into 1-inch segments	¾	cup fine cracker crumbs
	Salt	6	slices white bread, toasted

Alternate the lamb and the pineapple on skewers. Sprinkle lightly with salt. Dip in the margarine. Roll in the crumbs. Place under the broiler, preheated to 350 degrees, and cook for ten to twenty-eight minutes, until lamb is tender, turning the skewers often. Serve on toast.

Yield: 6 servings

Lamb Mousse

1	cup leftover lean lamb	¾	cup milk
1	envelope unflavored gelatin	¼	cup heavy cream or evaporated milk
¼	cup cold water		Salt
2	egg yolks, slightly beaten		Mint jelly

Put the lamb through a meat grinder. Soften the gelatin in the water. Combine the egg yolks and the milk in the top of a double boiler. Cook until thickened. Remove from the heat. Add the softened gelatin. Stir until the gelatin is completely dissolved. Add the ground lamb. Cool. Whip the cream until it is stiff. Fold into the lamb mixture. Salt to taste. Pour into a lightly greased one-pint mold. Chill until firm. Serve with mint jelly.

Yield: 5 to 6 servings

Liver-Steak Loaf

¾	pound beef liver, braised and ground	1	tablespoon chopped parsley
½	pound ground round steak	¼	teaspoon allspice
1	egg, lightly beaten	1	teaspoon salt
1	cup milk	1	tablespoon margarine, melted
1	cup soft white bread crumbs		Special Tomato Sauce (page 126)

Mix together all the ingredients except the sauce. Blend well. Form into a loaf. Arrange in a well-greased medium casserole. Bake at 350 degrees for one hour. Serve with the sauce.

Yield: 4 to 6 servings

Papa's Eye Round Roast

1	five-pound to eight-pound eye round of beef	Salt

Preheat the oven to 500 degrees. Sprinkle the meat with salt to taste. Place it on the rack of a shallow roasting pan. Roast, allowing four or five minutes per pound. At the end of the required time turn off the heat. Do not open the oven door. Let the roast remain in the oven for another one and one-half or two hours. The meat should then be brown on the outside and juicy inside. If it seems too cool when removed from the oven, reheat the oven briefly and warm the roast before slicing it.

Yield: 8 to 10 servings

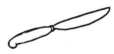

Roast Leg of Lamb with Vegetables

4	tablespoons lemon juice	2	cups fresh green peas
1	six-pound leg of lamb	10	small new potatoes, unpeeled
	Salt		Parsley butter
	Thyme		
2	four-ounce cans mushrooms		

Brush half the lemon juice on the lamb. Sprinkle with salt to taste and thyme. Place the lamb on the rack of a shallow roasting pan. Do not cover. Roast at 325 degrees allowing twenty-five to thirty minutes a pound for medium-done meat. After an hour, brush the remainder of the lemon juice on the lamb. When the lamb is almost finished, heat the mushrooms in a small saucepan and drain. Cook the green peas separately for ten to fifteen minutes, or until they are tender. Boil the potatoes and peel them after cooking. Serve the lamb on a heated platter encircled with parsley-buttered potatoes. Serve the green peas over the mushrooms in a separate serving dish.

Yield: 6 to 8 servings

Scrambled Eggs and Brains

¼	pound veal, pork, lamb or beef brains	¾	teaspoon salt
1½	teaspoons lemon juice	2	eggs, beaten
		1	tablespoon milk

Cover the brains with cold water. Add the lemon juice. Soak for thirty minutes. Drain. Remove any fiber or fatty membrane. Cover the brains with water. Add one-half teaspoon of the salt. Simmer gently for twenty-five minutes. Drain. Chop or put through the meat grinder. Set aside. Combine the eggs, milk, and the remaining salt. Add the brains to this mixture. Cook in the top of a double boiler, stirring, as you would to scramble eggs.

Yield: 3 servings

Turkey-Mushroom Soufflé

3	tablespoons margarine	2	cups cooked turkey
3	tablespoons flour	1	four-ounce can mushrooms, drained
¾	cup milk		
5	eggs, separated	¼	teaspoon cream of tartar
½	teaspoon salt	1	additional egg white
1	tablespoon finely chopped parsley		

Preheat the oven to 350 degrees. Combine the margarine and the flour in a saucepan. Whisk over medium heat until smooth. Add the milk gradually, whisking until the mixture thickens. Beat the egg yolks. Add the salt, parsley, and beaten yolks to the white sauce, whisking until well blended. Grind the turkey and the mushrooms. Mix with the sauce. Remove from the heat. Add the cream of tartar to the egg whites. Beat until stiff. Fold into the turkey mixture. Pour into a six-cup soufflé dish. Bake until brown and puffed.

Yield: 6 servings

Vegetables

Vegetables permitted in the bland diet for peptic ulcer are in two categories. The first consists of vegetables to be used during early convalescence. These must be mashed, puréed, or strained. They include asparagus, green peas, carrots, green beans, beets, and spinach.

The second group of vegetables, to be served as the patient progresses, need not be mashed, puréed, or strained, and are not limited to the foregoing six. Excluded are certain vegetables notably difficult to digest. (See the list of vegetables that are "permitted" and "not permitted" on page 29.)

The doctor decrees when the patient may advance to the second category of vegetables. However, the method of food preparation used during early convalescence may be continued in the more sophisticated recipes that follow if the patient finds that mashed, puréed, or strained vegetables provide greater comfort.

When the second category of vegetables is permitted, the ulcer patient may, with the doctor's sanction, enjoy finely shredded lettuce and diced tomatoes (skin and seeds removed).

Asparagus Special

7 canned asparagus tips	1 slice buttered white toast
	Egg Sauce (page 125)

Heat and drain the asparagus tips. Serve on the toast. Cover generously with the sauce.

Yield: 1 serving

Baked Acorn Squash

| 1 acorn squash | 1 tablespoon margarine |
| Salt | 2 tablespoons maple syrup |

Cut the squash in half crosswise. Remove the seeds and the stringy fiber. Bake, upside down, in a shallow baking dish at 350 degrees, for about forty-five minutes. Turn the squash halves cutside-up. Salt lightly. Melt the margarine. Combine with the syrup. Pour into the squash cavities. Bake for another twenty minutes, or until the squash is soft.

Yield: 2 servings

Baked Mushrooms

1½ pounds large mushroom caps	2 tablespoons margarine
1 teaspoon salt	½ cup light cream (or evaporated milk)
Cinnamon	

Place the mushrooms in a shallow baking dish. Season with the salt and a dash of cinnamon. Dab with the margarine. Add the cream. Bake at 400 degrees for about ten minutes.

Yield: 6 servings

Baked Potato, Beekman

| 1 baking potato | Salt |
| 3 tablespoons creamed cottage cheese | Paprika |

Scrub and dry the potato. Bake at 375 degrees for one hour or until done. Remove a slice from the top. Pile the cheese on the potato. Add a dash of salt. Sprinkle lightly with paprika.

Yield: 1 serving

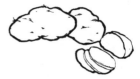

Tomato Casserole

2	cups canned tomatoes, strained	½	cup cornflake crumbs
¼	teaspoon salt	1	tablespoon margarine, melted
2	tablespoons sugar	½	cup grated mild
	Dash of allspice		American cheese

Combine the tomatoes, salt, sugar, and allspice in a greased medium casserole. Cover with the crumbs. Drizzle the margarine over all. Sprinkle with the cheese. Bake at 350 degrees for twenty-five minutes.

Yield: 4 to 5 servings

Corn Casserole

1	egg, beaten	2	cups canned cream-style corn, strained
1	tablespoon sugar		
¼	teaspoon salt	2	teaspoons margarine, melted
1	cup soft white bread crumbs	½	cup grated mild American cheese
½	cup milk		

Combine the egg, sugar, salt, crumbs, and milk. Add to the corn. Mix thoroughly. Pour into a greased medium casserole. Top with the margarine and the cheese. Bake at 350 degrees for thirty minutes.

Yield: 6 servings

Green Bean Bake

2	ten-ounce packages frozen whole green beans	1	cup sour cream
		2	tablespoons margarine
1	sprig parsley, finely chopped	1	cup soft white bread crumbs

Cook the green beans according to the package directions. Strain. Sprinkle with the parsley. Place in a greased medium baking dish. Top with the sour cream. Melt the margarine in a small saucepan. Add the crumbs and toss to coat well. Sprinkle over the sour cream. Bake at 350 degrees for twenty minutes, or until the crumbs are golden.

Yield: 6 servings

Green Beans with Cheese Sauce

1 ten-ounce package frozen green beans	1 cup Cheese Sauce (page 124) Mace

Cook the green beans according to the package directions. Strain. Prepare the sauce. Add to the green beans. Sprinkle lightly with mace.

Yield: 4 to 5 servings

Scalloped Corn

2 cups canned cream-style corn, strained	½ teaspoon salt
1 cup milk	¼ teaspoon mace
1 egg, beaten	1 tablespoon margarine, melted
1½ cups soft white bread crumbs	

Heat the corn. Add the milk. Stir in the egg, one cup of the crumbs, salt and mace. Pour into a greased medium baking dish. Combine the remaining ½ cup of crumbs with the margarine. Spread over the contents of the baking dish. Bake at 350 degrees for twenty-five minutes.

Yield: 5 servings

Scalloped Potatoes

6 medium potatoes	4 tablespoons margarine
½ teaspoon salt	1½ cups milk
2 tablespoons flour	

Peel and thinly slice the potatoes. Arrange a one-inch layer of the potatoes in a greased medium baking dish. Sprinkle with salt and a small amount of the flour. Add bits of the margarine. Repeat layering until all the ingredients except the milk have been used. Pour the milk over the contents of the baking dish. Cover and bake at 350 degrees until the potatoes are soft when pierced with a fork. This takes from one to one and a half hours. Remove the baking dish cover during the last fifteen minutes to brown the top.

Yield: 5 to 6 servings

Simple Summer Squash

1 medium summer squash	Mace
1 cup Medium White Sauce (page 124)	

Cut the squash in small pieces. Steam, covered, over boiling water. When soft, push through a food mill or a strainer. Combine the squash purée with the sauce. Dust lightly with mace before serving.

Yield: 2 to 3 servings

Spinach Bake

1 ten-ounce package frozen chopped spinach	¼ teaspoon allspice
	Salt
1 tablespoon finely chopped parsley	¾ cup sour cream
	¼ cup grated mild American cheese
1 four-ounce can sliced mushrooms, drained	

Cook the spinach according to the package directions. Combine with the parsley, mushrooms, allspice, and salt to taste in a greased medium casserole. Bake at 325 degrees for fifteen minutes. Top with the sour cream and cheese. Bake for another ten minutes, or until the cheese has melted.

Yield: 4 servings

Spinach Cosmopolitan

1 quart spinach	3 eggs, well beaten
3 sprigs parsley	2 cups milk
Salt	Mace
3 tablespoons margarine, melted	1 cup grated mild American cheese

Wash the spinach and the parsley. Cook in a very small amount of salted water for ten minutes. Drain. Cut out the stems. Chop. Drizzle the margarine over the spinach and parsley. Mix well. Turn into a greased medium baking dish. Add the eggs to the milk. Pour over the spinach and parsley. Sprinkle lightly with mace. Top with the cheese. Bake at 350 degrees for twenty-five minutes, or until the cheese has melted.

Yield: 5 servings

Summer Squash, Florentine

1	twelve-ounce package frozen summer squash	1	teaspoon sugar
2	cups canned tomatoes, strained		Salt
¼	teaspoon allspice	½	cup grated mild American cheese

Prepare the squash according to the package directions. Combine the squash with the tomatoes, allspice, sugar, and salt to taste. Place the mixture in a greased medium casserole. Cover with the cheese. Bake at 375 degrees for thirty minutes, or until the cheese browns.

Yield: 4 servings

Sunday Carrots

6	young carrots	¼	cup water
¼	cup light brown sugar	¼	teaspoon maple extract
¼	teaspoon salt	1	tablespoon minced parsley
4	teaspoons margarine		

Wash and scrape the carrots. Steam, covered, over hot water until just tender. Slice the carrots into thin rounds. Place them in a greased medium casserole. Combine the sugar, salt, margarine, and water in a small saucepan. Bring to a boil. Simmer for eight minutes. Stir in the maple extract and parsley. Pour the contents of the saucepan over the carrots and mix well. Bake at 350 degrees for about twenty-five minutes, basting once after fifteen minutes.

Yield: 4 servings

Sweet Potato Soufflé

¼	cup margarine	½	teaspoon allspice
2	cups canned sweet potatoes, mashed	¼	teaspoon salt
		5	eggs, separated
1	cup sour cream	1	egg white
½	teaspoon cinnamon		

Keep the margarine at room temperature for one hour to soften. Preheat the oven to 400 degrees. Cream together the sweet potatoes, sour cream, and margarine. Add the cinnamon, allspice, and salt. Beat the egg yolks lightly. Blend into the mixture. Whip the egg whites until stiff. Fold into the mixture. Pour into a greased medium soufflé dish. Bake for thirty minutes.

Yield: 5 to 6 servings

Tomato Pudding

1	cup cooked white rice	1	cup Medium White Sauce (page 124)
½	cup canned tomatoes, strained	1	tablespoon margarine
½	cup grated mild American cheese	¼	cup soda-cracker crumbs
		¼	teaspoon salt

Alternate the rice, tomatoes, and cheese, in layers, in a greased medium casserole. Pour the sauce over the top. Melt the margarine. Combine it with the crumbs and salt. Sprinkle on top of the tomato mixture. Bake at 350 degrees for twenty-five minutes.

Yield: 4 servings

Yam Creole

8	yams, cooked	3	cups pineapple juice
1⅓	cups crushed pineapple (canned without sugar)	1	cup light brown sugar
		½	teaspoon salt
1	tablespoon lemon juice	6	tablespoons margarine, melted
3	tablespoons orange juice		

Peel the yams. Cut each into four lengthwise strips. Arrange in a greased medium casserole alternate layers of the yams and pineapple, drizzling the lemon and orange juice between the layers. Combine the pineapple juice, sugar, salt, and margarine in a medium saucepan. Cook to a thick syrup. Pour the syrup over the yams. Bake at 350 degrees for thirty-five minutes.

Yield: 8 servings

Fish and Shellfish

Baked Fillets of Sole

1	pound fillets of sole	½	cup milk
1	tablespoon lemon juice	¼	cup buttered soft white
⅛	teaspoon paprika		bread crumbs
¼	teaspoon salt	1	tablespoon finely
1	tablespoon margarine		chopped parsley
1	tablespoon flour		

Cut the fillets into serving pieces. Arrange in a greased, shallow medium baking pan. Drizzle the lemon juice over the fish. Sprinkle with the paprika and salt. Melt the margarine in a small saucepan. Blend in the flour. Add the milk. Cook the mixture, stirring constantly, until thick and bubbly. Pour the sauce over the fillets. Sprinkle with the crumbs and parsley. Bake at 350 degrees for thirty-five minutes.

Yield: 3 servings

Baked Flounder with Sour Cream

1	sixteen-ounce package	½	teaspoon salt
	frozen flounder fillets	1	teaspoon finely minced
½	cup sour cream		parsley

Thaw the fillets at room temperature. Preheat the oven to 350 degrees. Arrange the fillets in a single layer in a greased medium baking pan. Cover with the sour cream. Sprinkle with the salt and parsley. Bake, covered, for thirty minutes, or until the fish flakes with a fork.

Yield: 3 servings

Baked Halibut

2 pounds halibut steak
1 tablespoon margarine
¼ teaspoon salt

1½ cups milk
Cheese Sauce (page 124)

Rub the fish with the margarine. Sprinkle with the salt. Place in a greased medium baking pan. Pour the milk over the fish. Bake at 350 degree for forty-five minutes. Baste frequently. Serve with the sauce.

Yield: 4 to 5 servings

Festive Fish Pudding

3 pounds haddock
½ cup white rice, cooked
1 tablespoon margarine
1 teaspoon salt

2½ cups milk
2 eggs, well beaten
Paprika

Poach the fish in salted water for about forty-five minutes, or until tender. Drain, skin, pick out the bones, and flake. Scatter a layer of the rice in a two-quart casserole. Add a layer of the fish. Season with the margarine and salt. Continue with alternate layers until the casserole is two-thirds full. Add the milk to the eggs. Pour this combination over the rice and fish. Sprinkle lightly with paprika. Bake uncovered for one hour at 350 degrees.

Yield: 6 servings

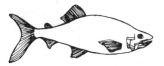

Fish Soufflé

5 tablespoons margarine	2 cups cooked fish
5 tablespoons flour	4 eggs, separated
1¾ cups milk	Special Tomato Sauce
¼ teaspoon salt	(page 126)

Melt the margarine in a medium saucepan and stir in the flour. Gradually add the milk, stirring constantly. Cook until smooth and thickened. Add the salt. Flake the fish with a fork and add to the mixture. Remove from the heat and add the beaten egg yolks. Fold in the egg whites which have been beaten stiff but not dry. Grease only the bottom of a medium casserole and turn the mixture into it. Bake at 325 degrees for forty-five to sixty minutes or until an inserted knife comes out clean. Serve at once with the sauce.

Yield: 6 servings

Fish Timbale

1 cup cooked haddock	½ cup melted margarine
½ cup cooked sliced mushrooms (reserve the cooking water)	¼ teaspoon salt
	Mace
	Paprika
1 cup soft white bread crumbs	4 eggs, well beaten
2 cups milk	Special Tomato Sauce
	(page 126)

Remove the bones and skin of the fish. Grind the fish and mushrooms in the blender, adding the water in which the mushrooms were cooked. Set aside in a large bowl. Cook the crumbs in the milk for ten minutes. Remove from the heat. Add the margarine, salt, a dash of mace, and a dash of paprika. When this mixture has cooled, add it to the fish mixture, beating it with a whisk. Blend in the eggs. Spoon the combined ingredients into a greased six-cup mold. Cover with aluminum foil. Set in a deep baking pan. Place in the oven. Pour water into the pan to within an inch of the top of the mold. Bake for forty-five minutes at 250 degrees. Serve with the sauce.

Yield: 6 servings

Salmon Delight

1	envelope unflavored gelatin	1½	tablespoons margarine, melted
¼	cup cold water	2	tablespoons lemon juice
1	teaspoon salt	1	cup cooked flaked salmon
2	egg yolks, slightly beaten	1	avocado, peeled and sliced
¾	cup milk		

Soften the gelatin in the water for five minutes. Combine the salt, egg yolks, and milk in the top of a double boiler. Cook over hot water for six to eight minutes, or until thickened, stirring constantly. Add the margarine, lemon juice, and gelatin. Stir until the gelatin is dissolved. Remove from the heat. Fold in the salmon. Turn into a greased six-cup mold. Chill until firm. Unmold on a serving dish and circle the salmon with slices of avocado.

Yield: 5 to 6 servings

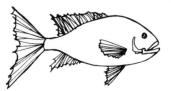

Sole au Gratin

1	one-pound package frozen fillets of sole	1	cup grated mild American cheese
	Salt		Soft white bread crumbs
1	tablespoon margarine		Paprika

Thaw the fillets at room temperature. When thawed, place in a greased medium baking pan. Sprinkle lightly with salt. Dot with the margarine. Bake at 400 degrees for twenty minutes. Cover with the crumbs and cheese. Lower the heat to 350 degrees. Bake for an additional fifteen minutes. The fish is cooked when it flakes with a fork. Top with a dash of paprika before serving.

Yield: 3 servings

Tuna with Macaroni

1	one-pound package shell macaroni	1	seven-ounce can water-packed tuna, drained
2	tablespoons margarine		
2	tablespoons flour	½	cup soft white bread crumbs
1	cup milk		
¼	pound grated mild American cheese		

Cook the macaroni according to the package directions. In a double-boiler top, over low direct heat, melt the margarine. Blend in the flour, add the milk. Stir in the cheese. Bring to the boiling point, stirring well. Place the double boiler top over hot water. Cook until the cheese is melted and the sauce thickened. Turn the tuna into the center of a greased shallow casserole. Mix the macaroni shells with the cheese sauce. Arrange around the tuna. Sprinkle with the crumbs. Bake at 375 degrees for fifteen minutes, or until the crumbs are browned.

Yield: 6 servings

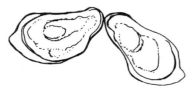

Baked Oysters and Noodles

12	ounces oysters	2	cups cooked broad noodles
¼	teaspoon salt		
¼	teaspoon allspice	½	cup buttered dry white bread crumbs
2	tablespoons flour		
1¼	cups milk		

Pick over the oysters. Remove any bits of shell. Cook the oysters in their own liquor until the edges curl. Add the salt and allspice. Remove the oysters from the saucepan, using a slotted spoon. Blend the flour with the oyster liquor. Gradually add the milk, stirring until the mixture thickens. Arrange half the noodles in a greased medium casserole. Cover the noodles with the oysters. Add the remaining noodles. Pour the sauce over the top. Sprinkle with the crumbs. Bake at 450 degrees for fifteen to twenty minutes.

Yield: 6 servings

Creamed Oysters

1 teaspoon lemon juice	3 slices white bread,
1 cup Medium White	toasted
Sauce (page 124)	Paprika
1 pint oysters	

Blend the lemon juice with the sauce. Pick over the oysters. Remove any bits of shell. Cook the oysters in their own liquor until the edges curl. Drain the oysters. Combine them with the sauce. Serve the creamed oysters on toast. Sprinkle lightly with paprika.

Yield: 3 servings

Luncheon Party Oysters

1 quart oysters	½ cup light cream or
3 tablespoons margarine	evaporated milk
3 tablespoons flour	2 egg yolks, slightly
¼ teaspoon salt	beaten
Mace	6 slices white bread,
	toasted

Pick over the oysters. Remove any bits of shell. Heat the oysters in their own liquor until the edges curl. Drain, reserving the liquor. Blend the margarine and flour in a large saucepan. Add the salt and a dash of mace. Add the oyster liquor gradually. Cook for five minutes, stirring until smooth and thickened. Add the cream slowly. Beat the sauce until it is glossy. Add the oysters. Heat. Add a small amount of the hot sauce to the egg yolks. Mix this combination well, then return it to the oyster mixture. Cook one minute longer, stirring constantly. Serve on the toast.

Yield: 6 servings

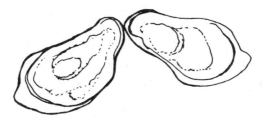

Salads

Avocado and Flaked Fish Salad

1	large avocado	2	tablespoons Cottage
1	tablespoon lemon juice		Cheese Dressing (page
½	cup cold cooked fish		130)

Halve the avocado. Remove the pit. Brush fruit with the lemon juice. Bone and, using a fork, finely flake the fish. Blend the fish with the dressing. Fill the cavity of the avocado with the mixture.
Yield: 2 servings

Cheesey Fruit Salad

3	tablespoons creamed cottage cheese, drained	3	stewed dried apricots Fruit Juice Salad
3	stewed pitted prunes		Dressing (page 129)

Mound the cheese in the center of a salad plate. Chop the fruit in small pieces. Spoon over the cheese. Serve with the dressing.
Yield: 1 serving

Cold Asparagus Salad (Ulcer-Diet Version)

8	canned asparagus tips Finely shredded lettuce leaf*	1	tomato, sliced and seeded, cut in eight wedges* Yogurt Sauce (page 126)

Arrange the asparagus tips on the lettuce nest. Encircle the lettuce with the tomato wedges. Spoon desired amount of the sauce over the asparagus.
Yield: 1 serving

*Check with doctor for permission to eat raw lettuce and tomato.

Cottage Cheese and Avocado Salad

1 large ripe avocado	6 tablespoons cottage
2 teaspoons lemon juice	cheese, drained
	2 stewed pitted prunes

Halve and peel the avocado. Remove the pit. Cut into cubes. Sprinkle with the lemon juice. Mash well with a fork or pastry blender. Mound the cheese in the center of two salad plates. Pile half of the mashed avocado on each cheese mound. Top each serving with a prune.

Yield: 2 servings

Festive Fruit Salad

1 cup boiling water	¾ cup canned peeled
1 three-ounce package	apricot halves, drained
strawberry-flavored	¾ cup canned crushed
gelatin	pineapple, drained
1 cup cold water	Fruit Juice Salad
	Dressing (page 129)

Add the boiling water to the gelatin. Stir until dissolved. Add the cold water. Chill. When partially thickened, fold in the canned fruits. (Reserve the juices for future use in a beverage.) Chill until set. Unmold. Top with the dressing.

Yield: 4 half-cup servings

Flaked Fish Salad

1 cup cold, cooked lean	2 tomatoes, skinned and
fish (haddock is a good	seeded, sliced thinly*
choice)	Salt
1 cup Yogurt Sauce (page	Lemon wedges
126)	
Finely shredded lettuce	
leaves*	

---

*Check with doctor for permission to eat raw lettuce and tomato.

Bone and flake the fish with a fork. Combine with the sauce, blending well. Arrange on lettuce beds on two salad plates. Circle each salad with tomato slices. Salt lightly. Serve with lemon wedges.

Yield: 2 servings

Mixed Fruit Salad (Ulcer-Diet Version)

1 cup canned crushed pineapple	1 banana
1 cup canned peach slices	Lemon juice
1 cup canned peeled apricot halves	Lettuce leaves, finely shredded*
1 cup canned pitted black cherries	

Combine the canned fruits in a medium mixing bowl. Chill. Immediately before mealtime, pour off the juices. (Reserve the juices for future use in a beverage.) Slice the banana in rounds. Sprinkle the slices with the lemon juice. Add them to the canned fruits. Spoon the fruits into a nest of finely shredded lettuce leaves, arranged in a salad serving bowl.

Yield: 5 servings

*Check with the doctor for permission to eat the raw lettuce.

St. Petersburg Salad

1 three-ounce package orange-flavored gelatin	½ cup pineapple juice
1 cup boiling water	½ cup cream, whipped
½ cup orange juice	1 banana
	6 marshmallows, diced

Dissolve the gelatin in the water. Add the juices. Chill. When the gelatin begins to thicken, stir in the cream, the banana (sliced in rounds), and the marshmallows. Refrigerate until serving time.

Yield: 4 servings

Tanta's Potato Salad

6 medium potatoes,
    unpeeled
1¼ cups Sour Cream
    Dressing (page 130)
    Salt

2 tablespoons finely
    chopped parsley
    Paprika

Cook the potatoes. Peel and slice. Mix with the dressing. Add salt to taste. Work in the parsley. Refrigerate. Sprinkle with the paprika before serving.

Yield: 4 to 5 servings

Desserts

Apple Bake

6 large apples
1 cup orange juice
1 cup heavy cream
¼ teaspoon cinnamon

1 tablespoon
    confectioners' sugar
¼ teaspoon rum extract

Pare, core, and cut the apples crosswise in one-quarter-inch slices. Arrange in a greased medium baking dish. Add the orange juice, 1/2 cup of the cream, and the cinnamon. Bake, covered, at 350 degrees for thirty-five minutes, or until the apples are tender. Whip the remaining cream. When it begins to stiffen, gradually add the sugar and rum extract. Continue whipping until stiff. Top the apples with the whipped cream.

Yield: 6 servings

Apricot and Cheese Treat

⅓ cup milk
½ teaspoon almond extract
2 tablespoons sugar
1 eight-ounce carton
    creamed cottage cheese

3 cups canned (peeled)
    apricot halves
6 teaspoons seeded
    raspberry jelly

Combine the milk, almond extract, sugar, and cheese in a large bowl. Blend into a smooth sauce, using a rotary beater. Drain the apricots. Spoon into a serving dish. Cover with the sauce. Dot spoonfuls of the jelly over the surface of the sauce.

Yield: 6 servings

Budget Rice Pudding

3	tablespoons white rice	¼	teaspoon salt
1	tablespoon sugar	½	teaspoon vanilla extract
1	quart milk		Dash of mace

Combine all the ingredients. Pour into a greased medium baking dish. Bake from one to two hours at 250 degrees. Stir several times. The pudding should not boil. The long, slow baking results in a creamy pudding with a delicious flavor.

Yield: 6 servings

Floating Island

2	cups milk	½	teaspoon vanilla extract
2	egg yolks	2	egg whites
	Salt	2	tablespoons
4	tablespoons sugar		confectioners' sugar

Scald the milk in the top of a double boiler. In a medium bowl beat together slightly the egg yolks, a sprinkle of salt, the sugar, and the vanilla extract. Add the hot milk to the egg mixture. Mix thoroughly. Return to the top of the double boiler. Cook over the hot water, stirring constantly until the mixture coats the spoon. Cool. Turn the custard into a large glass serving dish. Beat the egg whites until stiff. Gradually add the confectioners' sugar. Spoon the egg whites onto the custard. Chill thoroughly.

Yield: 5 to 6 servings

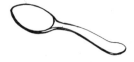

Freda's Fruity Dessert Treat

1	one-pound-one-ounce can fruit cocktail	¼	teaspoon salt
1¾	cups water	¼	cup orange juice
2	three-ounce packages black-raspberry-flavored gelatin		

Drain the fruit cocktail, reserving one-half cup of the syrup. Combine the syrup with the water in a medium saucepan. Bring to a boil. Dissolve the gelatin in the hot liquid. Add the salt and orange juice. Chill until the mixture mounds on a spoon. Fold in the fruit cocktail. Turn into a mixing bowl. Chill until firm. Serve in sherbet glasses.

Yield: 6 servings

Old-Fashioned Bread Pudding

2	slices stale white bread, diced	⅓	cup sugar
2½	cups milk, scalded	⅛	teaspoon cinnamon
3	eggs, beaten	6	teaspoons plum jelly

Soak the bread in the milk in a greased medium baking dish. Combine the eggs, sugar, and cinnamon in a bowl. Stir into the soaked bread and milk. Bake in a pan of water at 325 degrees for about forty-five minutes. When a knife inserted in the center comes out clean, the pudding is ready. Top each serving with one teaspoon of the jelly.

Yield: 6 servings

Peaches and Cream Dessert

6	slices True Sponge Cake (page 109)	¼	teaspoon vanilla extract
1	cup heavy cream		Canned peach slices, drained
1	tablespoon confectioners' sugar		

.Prepare the cake in advance. Whip the cream, adding the sugar and vanilla extract gradually. Continue whipping until stiff. Spread the whipped cream on the cake slices. Top each portion with several peach slices.

Yield: 6 servings

Peachy Scalloped Apples

1	teaspoon margarine	¼	cup dry white bread
3	peaches		crumbs
3	apples	¼	cup water
¼	cup light brown sugar		Whipped cream

Grease a medium baking dish with the margarine. Blanch the peaches. Slip off the skins. Slice in small pieces. Arrange half of them in the bottom of the dish. Pare and core the apples. Cut into eighths. Place half of the apples on top of the peaches. Layer the second half of the peaches over the apples. Place the remainder of the apples on top of the peaches. Sprinkle the sugar over the fruits. Cover with the crumbs. Pour the water over the contents of the dish. Bake, covered, at 250 to 300 degrees for thirty minutes. Remove the cover and bake for 15 minutes more. Serve hot in six dessert dishes with a dollop of whipped cream over each serving.

Yield: 6 servings

Plain Baked Custard

2	cups milk		Salt
4	tablespoons sugar	½	teaspoon vanilla extract
3	eggs		

Scald the milk. Mix the sugar, eggs, a pinch of salt, and the vanilla extract. Combine with the scalded milk. Pour into custard cups or a medium baking dish set in a pan of hot water. Bake at 300 degrees until firm. Test by running a knife blade into the center of the custard. When it comes out clean, the custard is ready to serve. Serve warm or chilled.

Yield: 2 servings

Rice Bavarian Cream

2	packages unflavored gelatin	⅔	cup cooked white rice
½	cup cold water		Salt
½	cup milk	½	teaspoon vanilla extract
3	tablespoons light brown sugar	⅓	cup heavy cream

Soak the gelatin in the cold water. Scald the milk in the top of a double boiler. Stir in the gelatin until it is entirely dissolved. Combine the sugar, rice, and a pinch of salt. Stir into the gelatin mixture. Add the vanilla extract. Whip the cream. Fold it into the rice mixture. Spoon into dessert dishes. Cool.

Yield: 6 servings

Rice Pudding

2	cups milk	3	eggs, slightly beaten
¼	cup margarine	½	cup cooked white rice
⅓	cup sugar		Cinnamon

Scald the milk. Add the margarine and sugar. Stir well. Add this combination to the eggs. Mix well. Add the rice and a dash of cinnamon. Turn into a greased medium baking dish. Bake at 300 degrees for about forty-five minutes, or until browned.

Yield: 6 servings

Tapioca Treat

1	quart milk	3	egg yolks, slightly beaten
¼	cup quick-cooking tapioca	1½	teaspoons almond extract
⅓	cup sugar	3	egg whites
¼	teaspoon salt	6	teaspoons quince jelly

Combine the milk, tapioca, sugar, and salt. Allow these to stand for five minutes. Add the egg yolks. Bring to a boil, stirring constantly. Remove from the heat. Add the almond extract. Beat the egg whites stiffly in a large bowl. Slowly stir in the tapioca mixture. Chill. Serve in sherbet glasses. Top each serving with one teaspoon of jelly.

Yield: 6 servings

Mamma's Pound Cake

½ cup shortening	1 cup milk
1 cup sugar	2 cups sifted cake flour
2 eggs	4 teaspoons baking powder
1 tablespoon almond extract	Mamma's Special Icing (page 130)

Preheat the oven to 350 degrees. In a large bowl mix together the shortening and sugar until creamy. Add the eggs and beat until blended. Add the almond extract. Add the milk and the flour alternately, mixing in three different additions. Beat at least three minutes. Add the baking powder. Mix one more minute. Grease and flour a nine-inch tube pan. Pour in the batter. Bake for thirty-five minutes, or until the cake tests done. When cool, ice with Mamma's Special Icing.

Yield: 6 to 8 servings

Mrs. Reiss's One-Egg Cake

2 cups sifted cake flour	1 teaspoon vanilla extract
2½ teaspoons baking powder	1 egg
¼ teaspoon salt	⅔ cup milk
⅓ cup shortening	Boiled Cake Frosting (page 131)
1 cup sugar	

Mix together and sift the flour, baking powder, and salt. Cream the shortening until soft and smooth. Gradually add the sugar, creaming until fluffy. Beat in the vanilla extract and egg. Add the flour alternately with the milk, beating until smooth after each addition. Turn into a greased eight-inch square pan. Bake at 350 degrees for about fifty minutes. When cool, ice with Boiled Cake Frosting.

Yield: 8 to 10 servings

One-Dish Specialties

Baked Cheese Omelet

1	tablespoon margarine	1	tablespoon finely
4	eggs		chopped parsley
4	tablespoons grated mild	¼	teaspoon salt
	American cheese		Paprika

Grease a shallow medium baking dish with the margarine. Beat the eggs. Add the cheese, parsley, and salt. Pour into the baking dish. Bake at 400 degrees for about fifteen minutes. Dust lightly with paprika before serving.

Yield: 2 servings

Baked Egg with Spinach

½	cup cooked spinach,		Salt
	finely chopped		Paprika
1	egg	¼	cup milk, approximately

Grease a custard cup or ramekin. Line with the spinach. Break the egg on the spinach. Add a sprinkle of salt and a dash of paprika. Add just enough milk to cover the egg. Bake at 350 degrees until the egg is firm, about fifteen minutes.

Yield: 1 serving

Baked Rice and Cheese

3	cups cooked white rice	1	cup milk, approximately
2	cups grated mild		Soft white bread crumbs
	American cheese	2	tablespoons margarine
½	teaspoon salt		
	Paprika		

71

Alternate a layer of the rice in a greased medium baking dish with a layer of the cheese. Season with a sprinkle of salt and a dash of paprika. Continue adding layers and seasonings until the dish is almost full. Add enough milk to come halfway to the top of the rice. Cover with the crumbs. Dot with the margarine. Bake at 350 degrees for twenty-five minutes.

Yield: 6 servings

Cheese and Carrot Bake

2 cups Mashed Carrots (page 145)
2 cups cooked white rice
2 cups grated mild American cheese

1 cup milk
2 eggs, beaten
1 teaspoon salt
Sprinkle of mace

Combine all the ingredients, but use only one and a half cups of the cheese. Mix well. Turn into a greased large casserole. Top with the remaining cheese. Bake uncovered at 350 degrees for one hour.

Yield: 6 servings

Cheese Fondue à la Riverhead

1 cup milk
1 cup soft white bread crumbs
½ teaspoon salt

1½ cups grated mild American cheese
3 eggs, well beaten

Combine the milk, crumbs, and salt in a medium saucepan. Cook over low heat, stirring constantly, until the mixture is smooth and bubbling. Remove from the heat. Add the cheese. Stir until well blended. Beat in the eggs. Bake in a greased medium baking dish at 425 degrees for fifteen to twenty minutes, or until golden brown.

Yield: 6 servings

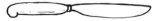

Cheese Soufflé

¼	cup margarine	¾	cup grated mild
¼	cup flour		American cheese
2	cups milk	5	eggs, separated
¼	teaspoon salt	1	additional egg white

Preheat the oven to 375 degrees. Combine the margarine and the flour in a medium saucepan, blending together over medium heat until smooth. Add the milk and salt. Cook until thick and smooth. Stir in the cheese, whisking until the mixture is smooth. Remove from the heat. Whisk in the egg yolks. Set aside. Beat the egg whites until they are stiff. (Use of a whisk for this procedure is recommended because the whites are more thoroughly aerated than when done with an electric beater.) Fold the egg whites into the cheese mixture, using a rubber spatula. Pour into a six-cup soufflé dish greased (unless directions at purchase indicate greasing is unnecessary). Bake for thirty-five to forty-five minutes, when the soufflé should be puffy and brown. Serve immediately.

    Yield: 6 servings

Easiest Rarebit

1½	cups Cream of Mushroom Soup (page 37)	1	tablespoon very finely chopped parsley
1	cup grated mild American cheese	4	slices day-old white bread, toasted
			Paprika

Pour the soup into a saucepan. Heat slowly to the boiling point. Add the cheese and parsley. Reduce the heat. Simmer, stirring constantly, until the cheese is smoothly melted. Spoon over the toast. Dust lightly with paprika.

    Yield: 2 servings

Egg and Cheese Timbales

1	cup warm milk	¼	teaspoon salt
½	cup grated mild American cheese	4	eggs, lightly beaten
⅛	teaspoon paprika		Special Tomato Sauce (page 126)

73

Add the milk, cheese, paprika, and salt to the eggs. Grease six custard cups. Fill with the mixture. Set in a baking pan half-filled with boiling water. Bake at 325 degrees until the egg is set. Turn out carefully onto hot dishes. Serve with the sauce.

Yield: 6 servings

Egg and Potato Bake

2	tablespoons margarine	3	medium potatoes, cooked and sliced
2	tablespoons flour		
1	cup milk	3	hard-boiled eggs, sliced
¼	teaspoon salt	¼	pound mushrooms, sliced
1	cup grated mild American cheese		

Melt the margarine in a medium saucepan. Blend in the flour. Stir in the milk gradually and bring to a boil, stirring until thickened. Add the salt. Stir in the cheese until it melts. Layer half the potatoes and half the eggs in a greased medium casserole. Top with half the sauce. Repeat the layers, adding the mushrooms to the remainder of the sauce before pouring it over the casserole. Bake at 350 degrees for twenty minutes.

Yield: 4 servings

Macaroni Pouf

½	cup small elbow macaroni	3	eggs, separated
1½	cups milk	1	cup soft white bread crumbs
6	ounces mild American cheese, grated	1	tablespoon finely chopped parsley
3	tablespoons margarine	⅛	teaspoon cream of tartar

Cook the macaroni in boiling salted water until tender. Drain. In a medium saucepan, combine the milk, cheese, and margarine. Cook, stirring constantly, over low heat until the cheese melts. Beat the egg yolks in a small bowl. Pour a little of the hot cheese mixture into the beaten yolks. Return to the hot cheese mixture. Blend well. Add the macaroni, crumbs, and parsley. Beat the egg whites and the cream of tartar, using a whisk, until stiff peaks form. Fold the beaten egg whites into the macaroni mixture. Pour into a greased large soufflé dish. Bake at 325 degrees for one hour, or until set.

Yield: 6 servings

Macaroni-Tomato Loaf

2 cups cooked macaroni
¾ cup finely diced mild American cheese
1 cup day-old white bread crumbs
1 teaspoon salt
½ teaspoon paprika

1 tablespoon finely chopped parsley
2 tablespoons margarine, melted
1½ cups canned tomatoes, strained

Mix all the ingredients together. Blend thoroughly. Turn into a greased large loaf pan. Bake at 350 degrees for about forty-five minutes.

Yield: 6 servings

Mushroom Soufflé

3 tablespoons margarine
3 tablespoons flour
¼ teaspoon salt
1 cup hot milk

½ teaspoon mace
3 eggs, separated
1 cup cooked mushrooms, puréed

Melt the margarine in a medium saucepan. Stir in the flour and salt. When smoothly blended, add the milk and mace. Cook, stirring constantly, until the sauce is thick and smooth. Remove from the heat. Beat the egg yolks lightly. Add to the sauce. Mix well. Spoon in the puréed mushrooms. Whisk the egg whites until stiff peaks arise. Fold into the mushroom mixture, using a rubber spatula. Turn into a greased one-quart soufflé dish. Bake at 350 degrees until puffy and brown. Serve immediately.

Yield: 5 to 6 servings

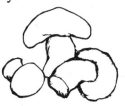

Noodle Ring

1	eight-ounce package medium noodles	½	teaspoon salt
3	eggs, separated	1½	cups Medium White Sauce (page 124)
½	cup milk	2	four-ounce cans button mushrooms, drained
½	cup light cream		
¼	cup grated mild American cheese		

Cook the noodles according to the package directions. Beat the egg yolks in a large bowl until they are thick and light. Add the milk, cream, noodles, cheese, and salt. Beat the egg whites until they are stiff. Fold the egg whites into the noodle mixture. Turn the mixture into a well-greased eight-inch ring mold set in a pan of water. Bake at 350 degrees for about one hour. Prepare the white sauce in a medium saucepan. Add the mushrooms. Stir constantly while heating to prevent sticking. Turn the noodle ring out on a round serving plate. Fill with the creamed mushrooms.

Yield: 6 servings

Parsleyed Green Peas and Mashed Potatoes

1½	cups puréed green peas	6	medium potatoes
2	tablespoons margarine, melted		Milk
3	eggs, well beaten		Margarine
¼	teaspoon salt		Salt
			Parsley Sauce (page 125)

Blend the green peas, two tablespoons of margarine, eggs, and one-quarter teaspoon salt. Pour into six greased four-ounce custard cups. Set in a baking pan containing hot water. Bake at 325 degrees for about thirty-five minutes, or until firm. Meanwhile, prepare the sauce. Peel, boil, and mash the potatoes, adding milk, margarine, and salt to taste. Beat until light and fluffy. Make wells of the mashed potatoes in the center of six luncheon plates. Unmold the green peas. Set in the potato wells. Pour some sauce over each serving.

Yield: 6 servings

Potato Gnocchi

2	pounds potatoes, peeled	2	quarts water
2	eggs, beaten	½	cup margarine, melted
1	teaspoon salt	1	cup grated mild
3	cups sifted flour		American cheese

Cook the potatoes in boiling salted water until tender. Drain and toss over very low heat for two minutes to dry. Mash in a large bowl until smooth. Beat in the eggs and salt. Blend in the flour to make a soft dough. Cover the bowl and chill for one hour. Heat two quarts of water to boiling in a large kettle. Form the dough into small fingers. Drop them into the boiling liquid, a few at a time. Simmer for five minutes or until slightly puffed. Remove with a slotted spoon to a shallow baking dish. Drizzle with the margarine. Sprinkle with the cheese. Bake at 400 degrees for fifteen minutes, or until puffy and golden. Serve at once.

Yield: 6 servings

Suggested Daily Menus

1

Breakfast	stewed apricots
	strained oatmeal with cream and sugar
	2 zwieback
	Sanka with milk and sugar
10.00 A.M.	malted milk, 2 soda crackers
Lunch	Borsch, American Style (page 36)
	Potato Gnocchi (page 77)
	Mixed Fruit Salad (page 64)
	True Sponge Cake (page 109)
	weak tea (with sugar and lemon if desired)
4.00 P.M.	warm weak cocoa, 2 Social Tea crackers
Dinner	Roast Leg of Lamb with Vegetables (page 47)
	(green peas, mushrooms, potatoes)
	Old-Fashioned Bread Pudding (page 67)
10.00 P.M.	Ovaltine with animal crackers

Breakfast	Cream of Wheat with milk and brown sugar
	2 eggs, scrambled in top of double boiler
	1 slice white toast
	1 glass orange juice and water (equal parts)
10.00 A.M.	banana and milk whip (blender)
	2 soda crackers
Lunch	Cream of Mushroom and Spinach Soup (page 37)
	croutons—1 slice day-old white bread, in small cubes
	Baked Chicken Breast (cold slices) (page 43)
	Tanta's Potato Salad (page 65)
	vanilla junket
4.00 P.M.	malted milk, 2 sugar cookies
Dinner	Liver-Steak Loaf (page 47)
	Tomato Casserole (page 51)
	Sunday Carrots (page 54)
	1 slice white toast and margarine
	New England Apricot pudding (page 159)
	Simple Uncooked Frosting (page 132)
	Sanka with milk
10.00 P.M.	warm weak cocoa topped with marshmallow cream

3

Breakfast	1 glass apricot nectar
	cornflakes with milk and sugar
	Baked Cheese Omelet (page 71)
	1 slice white toast
10.00 A.M.	malted milk, 2 soda crackers
Lunch	Cream of Spinach Soup (page 34)
	Baked Rice and Cheese (page 71)
	sliced tomato with skin and seeds removed
	Mrs. Reiss's One-Egg Cake (page 70)
	weak tea (with sugar and lemon if desired)
4.00 P.M.	flavored yogurt, 1 carton
Dinner	Sutton Place Sweetbreads (with green peas and mashed potatoes) (page 45)
	Scalloped Corn (page 52)
	1 slice white toast

margarine
Budget Rice Pudding (page 66)
Sanka and milk
10.00 P.M.   warm weak cocoa, 2 saltines

4

Breakfast   canned black cherries
Cream of Rice cereal with milk and sugar
2 slices white toast with margarine and grape jelly
warm weak cocoa
10.00 A.M.   buttermilk, 1 rusk
Lunch   Oyster Soup Special (page 37)
(with oysterette crackers)
Macaroni-Tomato Loaf (page 75)
Apricot and Cheese Treat (page 65)
weak tea
4.00 P.M.   1 glass apple juice, 2 sugar cookies
Dinner   Baked Halibut (page 57)
Parsleyed Potatoes (page 94)
Spinach Cosmopolitan (page 53)
Plain Baked Custard (page 68)
Sanka with milk
10.00 P.M.   warm milk, Melba toast

5

Breakfast   stewed prunes
Puffed Rice with milk and brown sugar
1 three-minute egg
1 slice white toast
Sanka with milk
10.00 A.M.   malted milk, rusk
Lunch   Avocado and Flaked Fish Salad (page 62)
Macaroni Pouf (page 74)
Simple Summer Squash (page 53)
Tapioca Treat (page 69)
4.00 P.M.   weak tea, 5 o'clock tea crackers
Dinner   Cream of Green Bean Soup (page 33)
Broiled Beef Liver (page 43)

79

10.00 P.M. Baked Mushrooms (page 50)
Corn Casserole (page 51)
1 soft roll with margarine
Baked Stuffed Pear (page 105)
warm weak cocoa topped with marshmallow

6

Breakfast sliced banana
Puffed Rice with milk and sugar
2 Parker House rolls with margarine and honey
Sanka with milk

10.00 A.M. 1 glass peach nectar, 2 zwieback
Lunch Vegetable Chowder (page 139) (with Pilot Crackers)
Easiest Rarebit (page 73)
St. Petersburg Salad (page 64)
Apple Bake (page 65)
Mamma's Pound Cake (page 70)

4.00 P.M. egg nog with rum extract, 2 vanilla cookies
Dinner Baked Fillets of Sole (page 56)
Stewed Tomatoes (page 95)
mashed potatoes
Mixed Fruit Salad (page 64)
Floating Island (page 66)

10.00 P.M. warm weak cocoa, 2 arrowroot crackers

7

Breakfast farina, milk and sugar with canned peaches
2 soft rolls, margarine and raspberry jelly
weak tea

10.00 A.M. buttermilk, Melba toast
Lunch Tomato Consommé, Jelled (page 32) (2 soda
crackers)
Cheese Soufflé (page 73)
Asparagus Salad (page 62)
Carrot Cake (page 108)

4.00 P.M. vanilla yogurt
Dinner Papa's Eye Round Roast (page 47)
mashed potatoes
canned green beans

1 slice white bread with margarine
Peachy Scalloped Apples (page 68)
Sanka with milk

10.00 P.M.   warm Ovaltine topped with whipped cream

4. The Bland Low-Residue Diet

The bland diet which the doctor may order for colitis or diverticulitis is a low-residue diet.

Medically, the suffix "itis" means "inflammation of." Thus, colitis means inflammation of the colon. There are several forms of colitis, which we need not go into here. The important thing to bear in mind is that the colitis patient for whom the doctor sees fit to order a low-residue diet will in all probability be greatly helped by adhering to it faithfully.

Diverticulosis is caused by small pouches—diverticula—which sometimes form along the walls of the colon, most frequently in older people. Diverticulosis is usually symptomless. It is actually a minor anatomical change in the body rather than an illness. However, when the diverticula become inflamed, diverticulitis ensues. In discussing the bland low-residue diet for this condition, we concern ourselves only with the dietary follow-up regime which the physician may order after acute periods of diverticulitis have been treated, usually in the hospital.

The bland low-residue diet is similar in most respects to the bland diet for peptic ulcer. The main differences between them are as follows:

The meal routine of the ulcer patient places emphasis on frequent meals, numbering as many as six a day. The low-residue routine usually calls for the classic three meals a day.

The low-residue patient is permitted soups containing meat or meat stocks. The ulcer patient is not.

Milk and milk products may be limited on the low-residue diet. This depends on the doctor's evaluation of each patient's needs. In the event that milk is restricted, soups, puddings, and sauces which include milk or cheese should not be used.

Spinach and squash, and all raw vegetables, are to be omitted from the low-residue diet.

All raw fruits are to be omitted from the low-residue diet. This includes the bananas and avocados which are permitted on the ulcer patient's diet.

Coffee and tea are permitted on the low-residue diet unless the doctor specifically rules out these beverages. Carbonated drinks—not iced—are also permitted on the low-residue diet.

Persons on the bland low-residue diet, in addition to using low-residue recipes, may also use bland ulcer diet and bland low-fat diet recipes, except those containing spinach or squash, raw fruits, or raw vegetables. Those whose milk intake is limited by the physician should not use recipes containing milk or milk products.

Soups

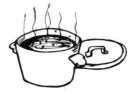

Beef and Barley Vegetable Soup

2 pounds soup bone (containing about one pound of meat)	1 cup cubed carrots
	2 cups cooked tomatoes
2 quarts water	1 cup fresh or frozen green peas
1 tablespoon salt	2 sprigs parsley, finely chopped
¼ cup pearl barley	

Pour the water into a kettle. Add the soup bone and salt. Cover tightly. Cook slowly for one hour. Add the barley and cook one hour longer. Cool the soup in the refrigerator. Skim off surface fat. Remove the soup bone. Cut off all fragments of meat and set aside. Add the carrots and tomatoes to the soup. Cook for twenty minutes. Add the green peas, parsley, and meat fragments. Continue cooking for fifteen minutes.

Yield: 10 to 12 servings

Beef Broth

1	pound beef, cut in small cubes	½	teaspoon salt
5	cups cold water	1	bay leaf
1	teaspoon finely chopped parsley		

Place the beef cubes in a kettle. Cover them with the water. Allow to stand for thirty minutes. Heat gradually to the boiling point. Add the remaining ingredients. Simmer, covered, for one to two hours. Remove the bay leaf. Cool. Skim off surface fat. Reheat before serving.

Yield: 4 servings

Beefy Mushroom Soup with Trimmings

1½	pounds soup bones, sawed or cracked by butcher	1	tablespoon zwieback crumbs
6	cups water	2	tablespoons water
1	teaspoon salt	¼	teaspoon thyme
½	pound lean ground beef	1	four-ounce can sliced mushrooms, drained
1	tablespoon minced parsley		

Place the first three ingredients in a four-quart pressure cooker. Cook for twenty minutes with the stem at the *cook* position. Let the stem return to the *down* position. Cool the soup stock in the refrigerator overnight. Skim off surface fat. Blend the ground beef well with the parsley, crumbs, two tablespoons water, and thyme. Form into small balls, using a one-half teaspoon measuring spoon. Pour the beef stock into a large saucepan. Heat to the boiling point. Add the meatballs. Cook, uncovered, for about fifteen minutes, or until they are tender but still firm. Add the mushrooms. Heat and serve.

Yield: 6 servings

Carrot Soup, South Bay

4	carrots	3	cups Beef Broth
2	potatoes		(page 85)
4	cups boiling water		Salt
			Soda crackers

Scrape the carrots. Grate coarsely. Peel the potatoes. Cut in thin slices. Cook the carrots and potatoes, covered, over low heat, until fork-tender. Lift from the cooking water with a slotted spoon. Push through a strainer or food mill. Return, puréed, to the cooking water. Add the beef broth. Salt to taste. Simmer for fifteen minutes. Serve with soda crackers.

Yield: 6 servings

Chicken Broth

1	three-pound to four-pound fowl, cut in pieces	1	teaspoon salt
		2	tablespoons white rice
			Mace
2	quarts cold water		

Place the chicken pieces in a large pot and cover with the water. Let stand for one-half hour. Heat slowly to the boiling point. Skim. Simmer gently, covered, for two hours. Add the salt and rice and simmer for about one hour longer. Remove the chicken pieces with a slotted spoon and reserve. Cool the broth and refrigerate for a few hours, or overnight. Skim the fat off the surface. Sprinkle the broth lightly with mace. Remove the skin from the chicken. Cut the chicken into small pieces and add to the broth. Reheat and serve.

Yield: 6 servings

Clam and Tomato Soup

2	cups clam broth	Paprika
2	cups tomato juice	Oysterette crackers
	Salt	

Combine the clam broth and the tomato juice. Add salt to taste. Chill. Serve cold in bouillon cups or cocktail glasses. Sprinkle lightly with paprika. Serve with oysterette crackers.

Yield: 4 servings

Lamb and Barley Broth

2 lamb shanks, trimmed	1 cup cooked tomatoes, strained
1 tablespoon salt	
2 quarts water	1 cup frozen green peas
¼ cup pearl barley	2 tablespoons minced parsley
1 cup cubed carrots	

Combine the first four ingredients in a large pot. Bring to a boil. Reduce the heat. Simmer for forty-five minutes. Add the carrots, tomatoes, and green peas. Cook for another twenty minutes, or until the vegetables are done. Cool. Remove the lamb shanks from the pot. Refrigerate the broth for several hours, or overnight. Skim off surface fat. Cut the meat from the shanks. Dice. Just before mealtime, return the meat to the broth. Add the parsley. Simmer for twenty minutes, stirring occasionally.

Yield: 6 servings

Raspberry Purée

1 ten-ounce package frozen raspberries	½ cup currant juice
	Mint leaves and confectioners' sugar (garnish)
1 cup water	
3 tablespoons sugar	
1 tablespoon quick-cooking tapioca	

Defrost the berries at room temperature. Simmer gently in a small saucepan for ten minutes. Press through a fine sieve. Discard the seeds. Combine the berry pulp, berry juice, water, sugar, and tapioca in a saucepan. Mix well. Bring to a boil over moderate heat. Remove from the heat. Add the currant juice. Cool and chill. Serve as a first course in sherbet or champagne glasses. Garnish with mint leaves frosted with confectioners' sugar. (The garnish is for eye-appeal only—not to be eaten!)

Yield: 4 to 5 servings

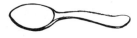

Meats

Baked Liver with Apples

1 pound beef liver, thinly sliced
2 large sour apples, peeled, chopped into small bits

Salt
½ cup water
Cinnamon

Preheat the oven to 350 degrees. Wipe the liver slices. Arrange in a medium greased casserole. Cover with the apple. Salt to taste. Pour water over this combination. Bake, covered, for about one hour. Serve with a sprinkle of cinnamon.
Yield: 4 servings

Blanquette de Veau (Modified)

1½ pounds veal
Boiling water
2 carrots, cut in quarters lengthwise
¼ teaspoon salt
1 tablespoon finely chopped parsley

½ pound fresh mushrooms, sliced
1 tablespoon margarine
1 tablespoon flour
2 egg yolks
1 tablespoon lemon juice
4 cups cooked white rice

Remove any fat or gristle from the veal. Cut the veal in cubes. Cover with boiling water. Let stand for twenty minutes. Drain. Place the veal in a Dutch oven or other sturdy cooking pan. Add the carrots, salt, and parsley. Cover again with boiling water. Simmer for one and a half hours. Add the mushrooms. Simmer for one-half hour longer. Melt the margarine in a separate saucepan. Add the flour. Stir in two cups of the veal stock. Simmer until slightly reduced. Beat the egg yolks in a medium bowl with the lemon juice. Add the hot veal stock gradually. Return the sauce to the pan. Stir until it begins to thicken. The sauce should be almost white. Pour the sauce over the meat and vegetables. Heat. Serve on rice.
Yield: 6 servings

Braised Tongue with Aspic Jelly

1 five-pound beef tongue
(fresh, not smoked)
Salt
1 teaspoon sugar
1 bunch parsley, finely
chopped

¼ teaspoon allspice
1 envelope unflavored
gelatin
1 cup cold water

Wash and scrub the tongue well in salted water. Simmer in fresh water until tender. Do not discard the water. Remove the skin. Place the tongue in a large stew-pan. Cover with the water in which the tongue was simmered. Add the sugar, parsley, and allspice. Simmer for two hours more. Remove the tongue and cut it into slices. Set aside the stock. Arrange the slices of tongue symmetrically in a large mold. Soften the gelatin in the cold water. Add the gelatin to the stock. Boil for two minutes, stirring constantly. Strain. Pour over the tongue. Chill in the refrigerator until the aspic is set. To unmold dip the mold in warm water almost to the edge. Shake the mold, cover with a plate, and invert.

Yield: 6 servings

Broiled Lamb Kidneys

2 lamb kidneys
Salt

Lemon juice
Lemon slices

Wash the kidneys. Split in half lengthwise. Remove the white centers and the tubes. Soak in cold salted water for thirty minutes. Drain. Pat dry with a paper towel. If the kidneys are very large, cover them with cold water and bring slowly to a boil before broiling. Drain. Brush the kidney halves generously with lemon juice. Cover the broiler pan with aluminum foil. Arrange the kidney halves on the foil. Place under the broiler preheated to 350 degrees and cook for ten to fifteen minutes, browning both sides. Serve on a hot plate. Garnish with lemon slices.

Yield: 1 serving

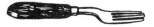

Chicken Soufflé*

1 cup milk	1 cup cooked chopped
3 tablespoons	chicken
quick-cooking tapioca	3 eggs, separated
1 teaspoon salt	¼ teaspoon cream of tartar
¼ cup grated mild	Paprika
American cheese	

Preheat the oven to 350 degrees. Cook the milk and tapioca in the top of a double boiler over rapidly boiling water for eight to ten minutes. Stir frequently. Add the salt, cheese, and chicken. Stir until the cheese is melted. Cool slightly. Stir in the well-beaten egg yolks. Whisk the egg whites until stiff, adding the cream of tartar. Fold in the beaten egg whites, using a rubber spatula. Turn into a greased medium casserole. Sprinkle lightly with paprika. Set the casserole in a pan of hot water. Bake for forty to fifty minutes or until the soufflé is delicately browned and firm in the center.

Yield: 6 servings

*Omit recipe if the doctor has limited the consumption of milk and milk products.

Escalloped Chicken and Noodles

1 five-pound chicken	1 six-ounce package
6 tablespoons margarine	noodles
4 tablespoons flour	1 cup soft white bread
1 teaspoon salt	crumbs
2 cups chicken stock	

Cook the chicken in a small amount of water until the meat drops from the bones. Remove and discard the skin and bones. Cut the chicken meat into large pieces. Make a sauce by melting four tablespoons of the margarine and blending it with the flour, salt, and chicken stock. Cook the noodles according to the package directions. Drain. In a greased large baking dish, arrange alternate layers of noodles and chicken. Pour the hot chicken-stock sauce over all to cover. Spread the crumbs over the top. Melt the remaining margarine and pour over the crumbs. Bake at 400 degrees for about twenty-five minutes, or until the crumbs are nicely browned.

Yield: 6 servings

Lamb Timbales

¼ cup Lamb and Barley Broth (page 87), heated and strained
2 eggs, slightly beaten
1 tablespoon margarine, melted
¼ cup soft white bread crumbs

1½ cups cooked ground lamb
Paprika
Special Tomato Sauce (page 126)

Stir the broth gradually into the eggs. Add the margarine, crumbs, lamb, and a dash of paprika. Turn the mixture into six well-greased custard cups or ramekins. Place the cups in a shallow pan containing hot water that comes to within an inch of their top edges. Bake at 350 degrees for about thirty minutes, or until a knife inserted comes out clean. Serve with the sauce.

Yield: 6 servings

Meat Loaf Special

½ cup zwieback crumbs
1 teaspoon salt
½ teaspoon allspice
1 tablespoon finely chopped parsley
2 eggs, beaten

½ cup cold Beef Broth (page 85)
¾ pound lean ground beef
¾ pound lean ground veal
Special Tomato Sauce (page 126)

Combine the crumbs, salt, allspice, and parsley. Mix the eggs with the beef broth. Add the crumb mixture and the egg mixture to the meat. Mix lightly with a fork. When well blended, shape into an oblong loaf. Place in a greased medium baking pan. Bake at 350 degrees for one hour. Top with sauce before serving.

Yield: 6 servings

Rock Cornish Game Hen Roast

2 Rock Cornish game hens
1 tablespoon minced
  parsley
1 cup pineapple juice plus
1 tablespoon Salt

2 tablespoons margarine,
  melted
1 tablespoon
  quick-cooking tapioca
2 cups hot cooked white
  rice

Place the hens in a large bowl. Combine the parsley and the cup of pineapple juice. Pour over the hens. Marinate for one hour. Preheat the oven to 400 degrees. Remove the hens from the marinade. Reserve the marinade. Pat the hens dry with towels. Salt them to taste. Coat with the margarine. Place in an ungreased large casserole. Bake uncovered at 400 degrees for thirty minutes. Heat the marinade. Pour over the hens. Cover the casserole and continue baking for thirty minutes longer. Remove the hens from the oven. Place on a serving platter. Surround with the rice and keep warm. Stir the tapioca into the tablespoon of pineapple juice. Blend into the marinade sauce. Cook until thickened. Spoon over the hens and rice.

Yield: 2 servings

Shepherd's Pie

2 cups mashed potatoes*
¾ cup canned diced carrots
¾ cup canned small
  green peas

Salt
1½ cups lean ground
  round steak

Preheat the oven to 450 degrees. Prepare the mashed potatoes. Combine the carrots and the green peas. Heat and drain. Arrange on the bottom of a hot greased medium casserole. Salt the meat to taste. Panbroil, without grease, in a hot iron skillet over which salt has been sprinkled. Turn the meat out over the vegetables. Cover the meat with the mashed potatoes. Bake for about fifteen minutes, or until the potatoes are browned.

Yield: 6 servings

---

*If the doctor has limited the consumption of milk and milk products, substitute a double portion of margarine for butter and omit milk in preparing the mashed potatoes.

Steak and Mushroom Casserole

1½ cups Beef Broth (page 85)
Salt
4 cube steaks

2 large potatoes, peeled and sliced very thinly
2 four-ounce cans sliced mushrooms, drained

Prepare the broth. Sprinkle some salt in an iron skillet or other sturdy pan. Panbroil the steaks, without grease, until they are about half done. Partially cook the potatoes, for about twenty minutes, in a small amount of boiling water. Preheat the oven to 350 degrees. Arrange the potato slices in the bottom of a greased two-quart casserole. Alternate the mushrooms and the steaks in layers over the potatoes. Pour a little of the broth over each layer. Bake, uncovered, for one hour.

Yield: 4 to 6 servings

Vegetables

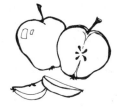

Baked Yams and Apples

½ cup dark brown sugar
½ teaspoon cinnamon
¼ teaspoon salt
3 cups canned sliced yams

3 cups peeled, cored, horizontally sliced apples
1 cup apple juice

Combine the sugar, cinnamon, and salt. Arrange the yams and apples in alternate layers in a greased medium casserole, sprinkling each layer with the sugar/cinnamon mixture. Pour the apple juice over all. Cover. Bake at 350 degrees for thirty minutes, or until the apples are fork-tender.

Yield: 6 servings

Boiled Asparagus

1 pound fresh asparagus	Simple Hollandaise
4 slices white bread, toasted	Sauce (page 129)

Use only the tips and tender portions of the asparagus. (Snap off the rough stems, scrub them with a brush, cut in small pieces, and use them for soup.) Cut the asparagus into one-inch pieces. Cook in boiling salted water to cover for fifteen to twenty minutes. Drain. Place on hot toast, and cover generously with the sauce.

Yield: 4 servings

Carrot Surprise

6 medium carrots	¼ teaspoon cinnamon
2 tablespoons light brown sugar	1 cup orange juice
1½ teaspoons cornstarch	2 tablespoons finely chopped parsley
¼ teaspoon salt	

Scrape the carrots. Cut in thin slices, crosswise. Steam, covered, over boiling water until just tender. Keep hot. Combine the sugar, cornstarch, salt, and cinnamon in a small saucepan. Stir in the orange juice. Cook until the mixture is thick and bubbly. Add the parsley. Boil for about two minutes, stirring to prevent sticking. Pour over the hot carrots. Mix well.

Yield: 4 servings

Parsleyed Potatoes

8 small potatoes, unpeeled	1 tablespoon finely chopped parsley
Salt	
¼ cup margarine	2 tablespoons lemon juice

Cook the potatoes, covered, in a small amount of salted, boiling water, until soft. Drain and peel. Melt the margarine in a medium saucepan. Blend in the parsley and the lemon juice. Stir, while cooking for about eight minutes. Add the potatoes. Roll them around in the parsley mixture to coat. Serve hot.

Yield: 4 servings

Party Green Peas

Sprig of fresh mint
½ cup orange juice
¼ cup sugar
1 eight and one-half ounce
   can green peas, drained

Liquid from the green
   peas (about 4 ounces)
Cinnamon

Cut the leaves off sprig of mint. Chop the leaves finely. Place in a small bowl. Bring the orange juice to a boil in a small saucepan. Add the sugar. Boil for one minute until the sugar is dissolved. Pour, steaming hot, over the chopped mint leaves. Cover with a saucer. Allow to steep. When cool, strain to remove the mint leaves. Place the green peas, their liquid, and a dash of cinnamon in a medium saucepan. Add the strained mint sauce. Heat and serve.

Yield: 2 servings

Stewed Mushrooms

1 pound mushrooms,
   sliced
   Beef Broth (page 85)
¼ teaspoon salt
   Mace

6 slices white bread,
   toasted

Place the mushrooms in a large, shallow skillet. Add enough of the broth barely to cover. Cover the skillet and stew the mushrooms for five to eight minutes. Uncover once or twice during the stewing process to stir the mushrooms around while they are cooking. Add the salt and a sprinkle of mace. Serve the mushrooms on the toast with a little of the stewing juice.

Yield: 6 servings

Stewed Tomatoes

8 large tomatoes
½ teaspoon salt

1 teaspoon sugar
½ cup cracker crumbs

Blanch the tomatoes in boiling water for one minute. Drain. Slip off the skins. Remove the stem ends. Cut in quarters. Cook, covered, in their own juice, or, if necessary, add a very small amount of water. Strain to remove seeds. Season with the salt. Add the sugar. Stir in the crumbs for thickening.

Yield: 6 servings

Yale Beets

1	sixteen-ounce can sliced beets	3	tablespoons sugar
1	tablespoon cornstarch	¼	teaspoon salt
¼	cup pineapple juice	¼	teaspoon allspice

Drain the beets reserving the liquid. Chop finely. Mix the cornstarch with one-half cup of the beet liquid. When smooth, gradually add the pineapple juice. In a medium saucepan combine the remainder of the beet liquid with the pineapple-juice mixture. Add the sugar, salt, and allspice. Cook until thick, stirring frequently. Add the beets. Reheat and serve.

Yield: 6 servings

Fish and Shellfish

Baked Fish

2½	cups canned tomatoes	2	sprigs parsley, finely chopped
1	four-ounce can sliced mushrooms, drained		Juice of ½ lemon
1	teaspoon salt	2	pounds fish (see note, top of page 97)
½	teaspoon paprika		Lemon slices

Preheat the oven to 350 degrees. Make a sauce by combining the first six ingredients in a medium saucepan. Simmer gently for fifteen minutes. Place the fish in a medium baking dish lined with aluminum foil. Cover with the sauce. Bake for about thirty minutes. Test for doneness with a fork. Flaking indicates that the fish is cooked. Garnish with the lemon slices to serve.

Yield: 6 servings
Note: Use striped bass, flounder, red snapper, haddock—not fat or oily fish such as salmon, lake trout, bluefish, mackerel, or butterfish.

Broiled Flounder Fillets

1 ten-ounce package frozen flounder fillets	2 sprigs parsley, finely chopped
¼ cup lemon juice	
Paprika	

Allow the fish to thaw at room temperature. Cut into serving pieces. Line a medium broiling pan with aluminum foil. Preheat the pan in the broiler for five minutes. Arrange the fish in the preheated pan. Combine the lemon juice, a sprinkle of paprika, and parsley. Drizzle generously over the fish. Broil about three inches from the heat just until the fish is nicely browned, brushing once or twice with the lemon juice-seasoning mixture. The precise cooking time depends on the thickness of the fillets.
Yield: 3 servings

Broiled Halibut Fillets

1 one-pound package frozen halibut fillets	2 sprigs parsley, finely chopped
Corn oil	1 lemon, thinly sliced
Paprika	

Thaw the fish at room temperature. Separate the fillets and cut them into serving pieces. Brush with the oil. Arrange the fillets in a shallow baking dish. Sprinkle with the parsley and paprika. Set the baking dish in the broiler about one inch from the heat source. Keep the source of heat low. Usually less than fifteen minutes will be needed to broil fish that is one-inch thick or less. When broiled in a baking dish, fillets need not be turned. Serve with the lemon slices.
Yield: 3 servings

Fancy Fillets of Sole

2	one-half pound fillets of sole	2	shelled oysters
	Salt	1	cup water
2	mushroom caps	2	egg yolks, beaten
		4	tablespoons margarine

Place the lightly salted fillets in a medium saucepan. Add the mushroom caps, oysters, and water. Cover. Bring to a boil and cook for seven minutes. Remove the fillets from the pan. Set aside cooking liquid. Place in a greased medium baking dish. Arrange a mushroom and an oyster on top of each piece of fish. Reduce the cooking liquid by stirring it over high heat. Remove from the heat. Add the egg yolks and margarine gradually. Season with salt to taste. Pour the sauce over the fillets. Place them under the broiler until they are delicately browned.

Yield: 2 servings

Fish-Vegetable Casserole

1	cup cooked fish	¾	cup water
1	ten-ounce package frozen mixed vegetables	½	teaspoon sugar
		½	teaspoon salt
1	fourteen-ounce can stewed tomatoes	½	teaspoon allspice
		¾	cup cooked white rice

Remove any skin or bones from the fish. Flake with a fork. Cook the vegetables according to the package directions. In a large saucepan combine the fish, mixed vegetables, tomatoes, water, sugar, salt, and allspice. Mix well. Bring to a boil. Simmer gently for five minutes. Put the rice in a greased two-quart casserole. Spoon in the contents of the saucepan. Cover and bake at 450 degrees for ten minutes.

Yield: 6 servings

Poached Halibut

1	quart hot water	1	two-pound to three-pound halibut steak
¼	cup chopped carrot		Special Tomato Sauce
2	sprigs parsley		(page 126)
1	teaspoon salt		

Put the water in a large kettle. Add the carrot, parsley, and salt. Boil for fifteen minutes. Wrap the fish in a piece of cheese-cloth. Place in the boiling water. Simmer gently, covered, for thirty to forty minutes, until done. Serve with the special sauce.

Yield: 6 servings

Tuna and Tomato Special

2 seven-ounce cans water-packed tuna, drained	½ teaspoon allspice
	½ teaspoon salt
	6 slices white bread,
2 tablespoons cornstarch	toasted
2 cups canned stewed tomatoes, drained	Paprika
	Lemon wedges
2 sprigs parsley, finely chopped	

Flake the tuna with a fork. Mix the cornstarch with a little cold water to make a liquid paste. Add to the tomatoes in a medium saucepan. Stir in the parsley, allspice, and salt. Cook until the mixture thickens. Turn the tuna fish into the tomato sauce. Mix well. Serve hot on unbuttered toast. Sprinkle with paprika. Arrange the lemon wedges alongside.

Yield: 6 servings

Five-Minute Paella

1½ cups cooked white rice	2 tablespoons finely chopped parsley
1 one-pound can whole tomatoes	Salt
	Sprinkle of mace
1 four-ounce can sliced mushrooms, drained	
1 seven-ounce can small oysters	

Combine all the ingredients in a medium saucepan. Cover. Bring to a boil. Simmer gently for five minutes or so.

Yield: 4 servings

Salads

Applesauce Delight (Low-Residue Version)

1 cup boiling water
1 three-ounce package
   black-raspberry-flavored
   gelatin
1 cup cold apple juice

¾ cup canned applesauce
   Mace
   Fruit Juice Salad
   Dressing (page 129)

Add the water to the gelatin. Stir until dissolved. Add the apple juice. Chill until the gelatin begins to set. Add the applesauce to the thickening gelatin. Sprinkle with mace. Pour into 4 sherbet glasses. Chill. Top with the dressing.
   Yield: 4 servings

Beet Salad

1 cup boiling water
1 three-ounce package
   lime-flavored gelatin
¾ cup cold canned beet
   juice
¼ cup cold water

1 cup canned sliced beets,
   finely chopped
¼ teaspoon salt
1 tablespoon lemon juice
   Orange Sauce (page 128)

Add the boiling water to the gelatin. Stir until dissolved. Add the beet juice and the cold water. Chill until the gelatin begins to set. Fold the beets, salt, and lemon juice into the thickening gelatin. Fill four sherbet glasses with the mixture. Chill until set. Top with the sauce.

Yield: 4 servings

Cranberry-Pineapple Salad

1	cup boiling water	1	cup canned, crushed
1	three-ounce package		pineapple, drained
	lime-flavored gelatin	4	tablespoons apricot jelly
1	cup cold cranberry juice		

Add the water to the gelatin. Stir until dissolved. Add the cranberry juice. Chill until slightly thickened. Fold in the pineapple. (Reserve the drained-off juice for other use.) Pour into four sherbet glasses. Chill until set. Top with the jelly.

Yield: 4 servings

Fruity Mold Salad

1	envelope unflavored gelatin	1	cup grapefruit juice
½	cup orange juice	1	tablespoon sugar
¾	cup crushed pineapple, drained	¾	cup canned apricot halves, peeled
½	cup pineapple juice (drained from crushed pineapple)		Guava Jelly Topping

Soften the gelatin in the orange juice. Heat the pineapple juice, grapefruit juice, and sugar. When the boiling point is reached, and the sugar is dissolved, add the mixture to the softened gelatin. Stir until completely dissolved. Chill until slightly thickened. Add the pineapple and apricots. Rinse a six-cup mold with cold water. Turn the gelatin mixture into the mold. Chill until set. Unmold and top with the jelly.

Yield: 6 servings

Mixed-Vegetable Salad

1 envelope unflavored gelatin
½ cup cold water
1½ cups hot tomato juice
¼ teaspoon salt
1 teaspoon lemon juice

1 cup canned green peas and carrots, drained
4 tablespoons Currant-Orange Sauce (page 126)

Add the gelatin to the water. Heat in a small saucepan until dissolved. Pour into the tomato juice. Add the salt and lemon juice. Mix well. Chill. When slightly thickened, fold in the green peas and carrots. Pour into four custard cups. Refrigerate. Unmold when set and serve with the sauce.

Yield: 4 servings

Molded Tuna Salad à la Felicia*

1 envelope unflavored gelatin
¼ cup cold water
2 egg yolks, slightly beaten
¾ cup milk
1½ tablespoons margarine, melted

4 tablespoons lemon juice
1 cup flaked water-packed tuna, drained
Special Fish Sauce (page 126)

Soften the gelatin in the water for five minutes. Combine the egg yolks and milk in the top of a double boiler. Cook over hot water until thickened, about six to eight minutes, stirring constantly. Add the margarine, lemon juice, and softened gelatin. Stir until the gelatin is entirely dissolved. Remove from the stove. Fold in the tuna. Turn into a mold. Chill until firm. Unmold before serving. Top with the sauce.

Yield: 4 servings

*Omit this recipe if the doctor has limited the consumption of milk or milk products.

Pear and Cheese Salad (Low-Residue Version)*

1 eight-ounce package cream cheese Paprika	24 canned asparagus tips, chilled
4 canned pear halves, drained	

Remove the cheese from the refrigerator one hour before meal-time to soften at room temperature. Dip butter paddles into scalding water, then chill them in ice water. Cut cheese into four-equal slices. With the fingers, form each slice into a ball, keeping the bottom paddle still while making circles with the top paddle. (A serviceable but less perfect cheese ball can be made with a melon scoop, a sugar spoon, or the fingers.) Place one pear half in the center of each of four salad plates. Put a cheese ball in the core cavity of each pear half. Dust the cheese balls lightly with paprika. Drain the asparagus tips well. Arrange six of them on each of the four plates, radiating from the pear halves like the spokes of a wheel, with the tips toward the edge of the plate.

Yield: 4 servings

*Omit this recipe if the doctor has limited the consumption of milk or milk products.

Prune and Apricot Salad

¾ cup dried prunes	1 cup cold water
¾ cup dried apricots	Pink Lady Topping (page 129)
1 cup boiling water	
1 three-ounce package cherry-flavored gelatin	

Cook the prunes and the apricots separately according to the package directions. Remove the prune pits. Chop the prunes and the apricots into very small particles. Add the boiling water to the gelatin. Stir until dissolved. Add the cold water. Chill until the gelatin begins to set. Fold the chopped fruits into the thickening gelatin. Pour into four sherbet glasses. Chill. Add a spoonful of topping to each serving.

Yield: 4 servings

Yummy Raspberry Treat

2	cups fresh raspberries	⅓	cup sugar
	Water		Simple Uncooked
4	tablespoons		Frosting (page 132)
	quick-cooking tapioca		

Place the raspberries and 1 cup of water in a medium saucepan. Bring to a boil and simmer for ten minutes. Strain. Discard seeds. Add enough water to the pulp and juice to make two and one-half cups. In a medium saucepan mix the tapioca and sugar with the berry pulp and juice. Boil for eight minutes over medium heat, stirring constantly. Cool. Serve with the frosting.

Yield: 4 servings

Desserts

Aimee's Apple Whip

4	tart apples	3	egg whites
¼	cup confectioners' sugar		Cooked Orange Dessert
2	teaspoons lemon juice		Sauce (page 127)

Peel and core the apples. Cut into small pieces. Steam, covered, over boiling water. When soft, push through a sieve. Add the sugar and lemon juice. Whisk the egg whites until they are stiff. Fold into the apple mixture. Spoon into sherbet glasses. Chill. Serve with a teaspoon of sauce on each portion.

Yield: 5 servings

Applesauce Brûlée

8	ounces canned	1	tablespoon light brown
	applesauce		sugar
½	teaspoon cinnamon		

Pour the applesauce into two ungreased custard cups. Sprinkle with the cinnamon. Cover with the sugar. Run under the broiler. Serve immediately.

Yield: 2 servings

Apple-Zwieback Special

2 cups zwieback crumbs	½ teaspoon mace
3 large baking apples	2 tablespoons margarine
½ cup light brown sugar	

Scatter a layer of the crumbs in the bottom of a greased large baking dish. Peel and core the apples. Cut them into thinly sliced rings. Place a layer of apple rings on top of the crumbs. Combine the sugar and mace. Sprinkle the apples with this mixture. Dot with small dabs of margarine. Repat this layering process until all the ingredients have been arranged in the dish, ending with crumbs. Bake at 350 degrees for thirty-five minutes, or until the apples are fork-tender.

Yield: 6 servings

Baked Stuffed Pears

6 large pears	1 cup grape jelly

Peel and core the pears. Stand them, vertically, close together, in a baking pan. Fill the centers with the jelly. Cover the bottom of the pan with water. Bake, covered, at 350 degrees for about twenty minutes, or until the pears are tender.

Yield: 6 servings

Prune Snow Pudding

24 dried prunes	2 tablespoons apple juice
2½ cups water	6 egg whites, stiffly beaten
½ cup sugar	Pink Lady Topping (page
2 envelopes unflavored gelatin	129)

105

In a medium saucepan, mix the prunes, 1½ cups of the water, and the sugar. Cover. Simmer for about fifty minutes, or until the prunes are tender. Cool. Remove the pits. In an electric blender, purée the prunes with the syrup in which they were cooked. In a medium saucepan, mix the gelatin into the remaining water. Let stand for five minutes. Heat just to boiling to dissolve. Stir in the apple juice and prune purée. Pour into a large bowl and refrigerate, stirring occasionally, until mixture mounds when dropped from a spoon. Add the beaten egg whites to the prune mixture. Beat until well mixed. Spoon into eight dessert dishes. Refrigerate for three hours, or until serving time. Add a dollop of topping to each serving.

Yield: 8 servings

Banana Surprise

3	bananas, peeled	3	tablespoons light brown
2	tablespoons lemon juice		sugar
3	tablespoons margarine, melted		

Cut the bananas in half, lengthwise. Arrange in a greased, shallow baking dish. Drizzle with the lemon juice. Blend the margarine with the sugar. Brush the bananas with this combination. Bake at 375 degrees for about fifteen minutes.

Yield: 3 servings

Broiled Grapefruit

| 1 | grapefruit | 2 | stewed prunes, pitted |
| 2 | tablespoons light brown sugar | | |

Cut the grapefruit in half crosswise. Remove the seeds. Cut out the pithy center with a scissors. Loosen each section by cutting with a grapefruit knife, or any sharp kitchen knife, along the membrane and the skin. Sprinkle each half with the sugar. Place in a shallow pan below the broiling unit, so the fruit is about four inches away from the heat source. Broil for about fifteen minutes, or until the skin begins to brown. Garnish with a prune in each center before serving.

Yield: 2 servings

Broiled Peaches à la Ce-Ce

4	large ripe peaches	1	tablespoon lemon juice
1	tablespoon light brown sugar		Mace
		4	marshmallows

Blanch the peaches. Slip off the skin. Halve. Remove the pits. Place peaches, hollow side up, in a greased shallow medium baking pan. Sprinkle with the sugar and lemon juice. Dust lightly with mace. Broil for five minutes, or until tender. Set a marshmallow in each peach-cavity and serve immediately.

Yield: 4 servings

Cherry Tapioca

	Cherry juice	¾	cup light brown sugar
1½	cups canned sour cherries, drained		Dash of mace
2	teaspoons lemon juice	⅓	cup quick-cooking tapioca
1	tablespoon margarine, melted		

Add water to the cherry juice as needed to make 2½ cups of liquid. Combine all the ingredients in a greased medium baking dish. Mix well. Bake at 350 degrees for thirty minutes. Stir every ten minutes. Stir once more when removing from the oven. Serve warm or cold.

Yield: 6 servings

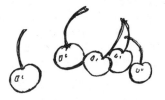

Carrot Cake, Keith Lane

2 cups sugar	4 eggs
1 cup vegetable oil	2 cups shredded carrots
2 teaspoons cinnamon	Simple Uncooked
2 teaspoons baking soda	Frosting (page 132)
1 teaspoon salt	
2 teaspoons double-acting baking powder	

Mix the sugar and the oil in a large mixing bowl. Beat with an electric beater until light. Sift together the remaining dry ingredients. Add, alternately with the eggs, to the sugar-oil mixture, beating well after each addition. Stir in the carrots with a wooden spoon. Bake at 350 degrees in a greased nine-inch tube or bundt pan for about one hour, or until the cake tests done. Simple Uncooked Frosting goes well with this cake.

Yield: 6 to 8 servings

Golden Glow Cake*

⅔ cup milk	2 cups cake flour
2 tablespoons margarine	2 teaspoons baking powder
4 eggs	⅓ cup frozen orange juice
2 cups sugar	concentrate, thawed
½ teaspoon salt	Quince Jelly Lemon
½ teaspoon orange extract	Icing (page 165)

Scald the milk. Add the margarine. Cool. Beat the eggs in a large bowl until thick and lemon-colored. Add the sugar gradually. Beat until light and fluffy. Add the salt and orange extract. Pour in the cooled milk mixture. Beat again. Sift the cake flour and baking powder together. Add to the batter alternately with the orange juice concentrate, ending with the dry ingredients. Beat thoroughly. Pour into three round eight-inch cake pans, which have been greased on the bottom and lined with waxed paper. Bake at 350 degrees for twenty-five minutes. Turn out onto wire racks. Remove the paper. Lemon Icing goes well on top of this cake. Quince Jelly as filling between layers.

Yield: 6 servings

*Omit this recipe if the doctor has limited the consumption of milk or milk products.

Pineapple Cake

½ pound margarine	1¾ cups sifted flour
1½ cups sugar	1 teaspoon vanilla extract
4 eggs	1½ cups crushed pineapple

Cream the margarine well in a large bowl, using a rotary beater on high speed. Add the sugar gradually. Continue to beat for ten minutes. Add the eggs, one at a time. Beat well after each addition. Add the flour and the vanilla extract on low speed. Drain the pineapple (reserving the juice for another occasion) and fold it into the batter. Pour the batter into an eight-inch tube pan, greased on the bottom and lined with waxed paper. Thump the bottom of the pan about ten times, while turning it, to level the batter and remove air bubbles. Bake at 350 degrees for forty-five to sixty minutes. Cool in the pan for ten minutes. Turn out onto a wire rack. Remove the paper.

Yield: 10 to 12 servings

Rita's Fruit Cocktail Cake

2 cups flour	2 cups fruit cocktail, drained
1½ cups granulated sugar	
2 teaspoons baking soda	½ cup light brown sugar
2 eggs	

Combine the first five ingredients. Mix well. Pour into a greased, floured eight-inch square pan. Sprinkle with the brown sugar. Bake at 325 degrees for forty to fifty minutes.

Yield: 8 servings

True Sponge Cake à la Theresa

1 cup flour	1 cup sugar
¼ teaspoon salt	4 teaspoons lemon juice
4 eggs, separated	

Sift the flour. Add the salt and sift again. Beat the egg yolks in a large mixing bowl until they are thick and lemon-colored. Add the sugar gradually and beat again. Add the lemon juice. Mix thoroughly. Beat the egg whites until stiff. Fold in the flour alternately with the egg whites. Do not beat the cake at this stage. Pour batter into a floured 17 × 11 × 1 inch sheet tin or ungreased 9½ × 5 × 3¾ inch loaf pan. For the sheet tin, bake at 325 degrees for thirty minutes. For the loaf pan, bake at 300 to 325 degrees for forty to sixty minutes.

Yield: 6 to 8 servings

One-Dish Specialties

Baked Eggs in Rice Nests

2	cups cooked white rice	Salt
4	eggs	Paprika

• Grease four custard cups or ramekins. Line with the rice. Break an egg into each rice nest. Add to each a sprinkle of salt and a dash of paprika. Bake, covered, at 350 degrees for about fifteen minutes, or until the eggs are firm.

Yield: 4 servings

Chicken with Mushrooms

1	four-pound fowl, cut in pieces	½	pound mushrooms, sliced
2	teaspoons salt	5	tablespoons margarine
6	cups broad noodles, cooked according to the package directions	2	cups hot chicken stock
		½	cup soft white bread crumbs

Wash the chicken pieces. Place in a large cooking pot. Add water to half cover. Simmer, covered, for two to three hours, or until tender. Add the salt after the first hour of cooking. When the chicken is tender, remove the meat from the bones. Place layers of half of the hot noodles, half of the chicken, and half of the mushrooms in a greased large casserole. Repeat the layers with the remaining amounts. Add three tablespoons of the margarine to the stock. Pour over the contents of the casserole. Cover with crumbs. Melt the remaining margarine and pour over the crumbs. Bake, uncovered, at 350 degrees for about twenty minutes, or until browned. (Note: The patient does not eat the chicken skin.)

Yield: 6 to 8 portions

Baked Jelly Omelet

2 eggs	1 tablespoon grape jelly
1 tablespoon water	¼ teaspoon confectioners'
⅛ teaspoon salt	sugar

Apply a generous amount of non-caloric, no-fat cooking spray to the interior of a small, shallow baking dish. Beat the eggs so yolks and whites are well mixed. Add the water and salt. Pour the eggs into the baking dish. Bake at 400 degrees for about fifteen minutes, or until firm on top. Place the omelet on a serving plate. Fold once and spoon the jelly inside the fold. Sprinkle the omelet lightly with the sugar.

Yield: 1 serving

Lima Bean Loaf

1 ten-ounce package frozen lima beans, thawed	½ cup cornflake crumbs
	½ cup crushed soda-cracker crumbs
1 egg, lightly beaten	3 teaspoons margarine, melted
2 tablespoons light brown sugar	Special Tomato Sauce (page 126)
½ cup tomato juice	
1 tablespoon lemon juice	

Mix well all the ingredients except the sauce. Form into a loaf. Bake in a greased large casserole at 350 degrees for forty-five minutes. Heat the sauce and serve in a separate sauce dish.

Yield: 5 to 6 servings

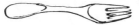

Homemade Fettucini Alfredo (Modified)

3	cups flour	6	quarts water
4	teaspoons salt	½	cup margarine, cut in
3	eggs		small pieces
4	tablespoons corn oil	2	cups grated mild
¼	cup cold water		American cheese*
	Cornstarch		

Sift the flour and two teaspoons of the salt together in a large bowl. Make a well in the center. Add the eggs, three tablespoons of the oil, and the cold water. Blend, using the fingers, to make a stiff dough. Turn out on a large pastry board. Add no additional flour. Knead for ten minutes, or until the dough is smooth and soft. Wrap in plastic wrap. Set aside at room temperature for one hour. Sprinkle the pastry board with cornstarch. Roll out the dough, a quarter of it at a time, to a very thin rectangle. Fold each rectangle into quarters lengthwise. Slice the dough into one-quarter-inch-wide strips. Unwind the strips. Let them dry on clean towels for one hour.

In a large kettle heat the water to the boiling point. Add the remaining salt and oil. Cook the fettucini for five minutes if "al dente" doneness (a slight resistance to the teeth) is desired. Cook a few minutes longer if tenderness is preferred. Drain well and turn out onto a heated serving platter. Add the pieces of margarine. Toss with a fork and a spoon until the margarine melts. Add the cheese— or substitute—if contraindicated. Continue to toss until the fettucini are coated and glistening. Never melt the margarine before adding it to the fettucini.

Yield: 3 to 4 servings

*Substitute tomato sauce for the cheese if the doctor has limited the consumption of milk or milk products.

Linguine à la Ruth

4	ounces linguine	2	cups Special Tomato
3	tablespoons margarine		Sauce (page 126)

Cook the linguine according to the package directions. Drain. Melt the margarine in a medium saucepan. Toss the hot linguine with the margarine. Heat the sauce and mix well with the linguine.

Yield: 2 to 4 servings

Macaroni and Cheese Timbales*

1½ cups cooked elbow macaroni	1½ cups milk
2 eggs, well beaten	Paprika
¼ teaspoon salt	Special Tomato Sauce
1 cup grated mild American cheese	(page 126)

Divide the macaroni among six greased custard cups. Mix together the eggs, salt, cheese, and milk. Pour over the macaroni in the custard cups. Set the cups in a pan of hot water. Bake at 350 degrees for thirty minutes, or until firm. Top with a dash of paprika. Serve with the sauce.

Yield: 6 servings

*Omit this recipe if the doctor has limited the consumption of milk and milk products.

Chicken Liver Delight

4 tablespoons margarine	1 hard-boiled egg, chopped
1 pound chicken livers	8 slices thin white bread, toasted
2 tablespoons lemon juice	
½ teaspoon salt	
Thyme	4 glasses tomato juice

Melt two tablespoons of the margarine in a medium saucepan. Add the livers. Cook, covered, stirring occasionally until they are no longer pink. Push through a food mill or a strainer. Melt the remaining margarine. In a medium bowl, blend the mashed livers, the melted margarine, lemon juice, salt and a dash of thyme. When thoroughly mixed, place in an ungreased two and one-half cup mold. Chill for several hours. Carefully unmold. Garnish with the chopped egg. Serve each portion on two slices of hot toast, each cut in quarters diagonally. Serve with tomato juice.

Yield: 4 servings

Rice Ring De Luxe

4 cups cooked white rice, hot
1 cup canned peas and carrots, heated and drained

2 tablespoons margarine, melted
1 pound cooked chicken, sliced

Combine the first three ingredients while they are hot. Mix well. Press the mixture lightly into a well greased medium-sized mold. Unmold on a warmed round platter. Serve with hot sliced chicken.

Yield: 6 servings

Skewered Scallops and Mushrooms

1½ pounds sea scallops
½ pound medium mushrooms
¼ cup melted margarine

4 tablespoons Simple Hollandaise Sauce (page 129)

Rinse and drain scallops. Cut in one-inch chunks. Alternate scallops and mushrooms on four slender skewers. Brush generously with margarine. Place skewers on a flat pan and put under the broiler four inches away from the source of heat. Baste continuously with margarine and turn once while broiling for five to seven minutes, or until the scallops turn opaque throughout. (This is determined by cutting a gash to test.) Top each serving with a tablespoon of the sauce.

Yield: 4 servings

North Shore Sweet Potatoes

5 cups sweet potatoes, cooked and mashed
½ cup honey
¼ cup pineapple juice
¼ teaspoon salt

3 tablespoons melted margarine
1 tablespoon lemon juice
1 pound breast of roast turkey, sliced

Combine the sweet potatoes with the honey, pineapple juice, salt, margarine, and lemon juice. Bake in a greased large casserole at 350 degrees for forty-five minutes. Serve with hot turkey.

Yield: 6 servings

Vegetable Loaf

½ cup green peas	½ teaspoon salt
½ cup green beans	½ teaspoon paprika
½ cup chopped carrots	1 egg
1½ cups tomato juice	2 cups Simple Hollandaise
1 cup soft white bread	Sauce (page 129)
crumbs	

Cook and strain the green peas. Cut the green beans in small pieces. Steam the green beans and carrots until barely tender. Combine the vegetables. Add to them the tomato juice, crumbs, salt, paprika, and egg. Blend thoroughly. Turn into a greased medium loaf pan. Bake at 350 degrees until firm. Serve with the sauce.

Yield: 6 servings

Suggested Daily Menus

1

Breakfast

1 baked apple, peeled and cored
Cream of Wheat with milk and
    sugar
2 slices white toast with
    margarine and honey

coffee (if permitted) with sugar
    and milk or cream

Lunch

Carrot Soup, South Bay
    (page 86)
Molded Tuna Fish Salad (page
    102)

soda crackers
Banana Surprise (page 106)
ginger ale (no ice)

Dinner

Shepherd's Pie (page 92)
(mashed potato, green peas,
    carrots)
Prune and Apricot Salad (see
    page 103)

1 slice white toast with
    margarine
Golden Glow Cake (page 108)
Lemon Icing (page 165)
tea (if permitted)

(IF DOCTOR LIMITS CONSUMPTION OF MILK OR MILK PRODUCTS)

Breakfast

1 baked apple, peeled and cored
1 small broiled lamb chop about
    1″ thick

1 slice white toast with
    margarine
black coffee (if permitted) with
    sugar

Lunch

Carrot Soup, South Bay (page
    86)
Skewered Scallops and
    Mushrooms (page 114)

Banana Surprise (page 106)
ginger ale (no ice)

Dinner

Poached Halibut (page 98)
Stewed Tomatoes (page 195)
Parsleyed Potatoes (page 94)
Prune and Apricot Salad (page
    103)

1 slice white toast with
    margarine
Golden Glow Cake (page 108)
Lemon Icing (page 165)
tea (if permitted)

2

Breakfast

1 glass canned orange and
pineapple juice (equal parts)
strained oatmeal with light
brown sugar and milk

2 poached eggs on white toast
    with margarine
coffee (if permitted) with milk
    and sugar

Lunch

Broiled Ground Beef Patty
    (page 40)
2 slices day-old white bread
Scalloped Corn (page 52)

Apple-Zwieback Special   (page
    105)
ginger ale (no ice)

Dinner

Blanquette de Veau (page 88)
(rice, mushrooms, carrots)
2 slices white toast with
    margarine

Pineapple Cake (page 109)
coffee (if permitted) with milk
    and sugar

(IF DOCTOR LIMITS CONSUMPTION OF MILK OR MILK PRODUCTS)

Breakfast

1 glass canned orange and
    pineapple juice (equal parts)

2 poached eggs on white toast
    with margarine
black coffee (if permitted) with
    sugar

Lunch

Broiled Ground Beef Patty
    (page 40)
2 slices day-old white bread
Marmalade Beets (page 145)

Apple-Zwieback Special   (page
    105)
ginger ale (no ice)

Dinner

Blanquette de Veau (page 88)
(rice, mushrooms, carrots)
2 slices white toast with
    margarine

Pineapple Cake (page 109)
black coffee (if permitted)

3

Breakfast
stewed peaches
2 soft-boiled eggs

2 slices white toast
tea (if permitted)

Lunch

Shell Macaroni with Tomato
    Sauce (page 126)
Fruity Mold Salad (page 41)

Rice Pudding (page 69)
ginger ale (no ice)

Dinner

Beefy Mushroom Soup with Trimmings (page 85)
Baked Liver with Apples (page 88)

baked potato with margarine
Baked Stuffed Pear (page 105)
Sanka (if permitted) with milk and sugar

(IF DOCTOR LIMITS CONSUMPTION OF MILK OR MILK PRODUCTS)

Breakfast

stewed peaches
2 soft-boiled eggs

2 slices white toast
tea (if permitted)

Lunch

Shell Macaroni with Tomato Sauce (page 126)
Fruity Mold Salad (page 101)

Carrot Cake, Keith Lane (page 108)
ginger ale (no ice)

Dinner

Beefy Mushroom Soup with Trimmings (page 85)
Baked Liver with Apples (page 88)

baked potato with margarine
Baked Stuffed Pear (page 105)
Sanka (if permitted)

4

Breakfast

stewed prunes and apricots
cornflakes with milk and light brown sugar
Baked Egg with Spinach (page 71)

1 slice white toast with margarine
tea (if permitted) with sugar

Lunch

Tuna and Tomato Special (page 99)
soft roll with margarine

Beet Salad (page 100)
Tapioca Treat (page 69)
ginger ale (no ice)

Dinner

Clam and Tomato Soup (page 86)
oysterette crackers
Broiled Flounder Fillets (page 97)

Baked Yams and Apples (page 93)
Broiled Peaches à la Ce-Ce (page 107)
coffee (if permitted) with milk and sugar

(IF DOCTOR LIMITS THE CONSUMPTION OF MILK OR MILK PRODUCTS)

Breakfast

stewed prunes and apricots
Baked Jelly Omelet (page 111)

1 slice white toast with margarine
tea (if permitted) with sugar

Lunch

Baked Fish (page 96)
soft roll with margarine
Beet Salad (page 100)

Cherry Tapioca (page 107)
ginger ale (no ice)

Dinner

Clam and Tomato Soup (page 86)
oysterette crackers
Broiled Flounder Fillets (page 97)

Baked Yams and Apples (page 93)
Broiled Peaches à la Ce-Ce (page 107)
black coffee (if permitted)

5

Breakfast

1 glass canned apricot nectar
corn meal with milk and sugar
1 egg scrambled in top of double boiler

2 slices white toast
tea (if permitted)

Lunch

Five-minute Paella (page 99)
Applesauce Delight (page 100)

True Sponge Cake à la Theresa (page 109)
ginger ale (no ice)

119

Dinner

Chicken Broth (page 86)
Rock Cornish Game Hen Roast
   (page 92)
rice, pineapple juice
Stewed Mushrooms (page 95)

Party Green Peas (page 95)
Rita's Fruit Cocktail
   (page 99)
coffee (if permitted) with milk

(IF DOCTOR LIMITS CONSUMPTION OF MILK OR MILK PRODUCTS)

Breakfast

1 glass canned apricot nectar
1½ Broiled Lamb Kidneys
   (page 89)

2 slices white toast
tea (if permitted)

Lunch

Five-minute Paella (page 99)
Applesauce Delight (page 100)

True Sponge Cake à la Theresa
   (page 109)
ginger ale (no ice)

Dinner

Chicken Broth (page 86)
Rock Cornish Game Hen Roast
   (page 92)
rice, pineapple juice
Stewed Mushrooms (page 95)

Party Green Peas (page 95)
Rita's Fruit Cocktail Cake
   (page 109)
black coffee (if permitted)

6

Breakfast

Broiled Grapefruit (page 106)
cheese omelet (2 eggs)

2 slices white toast with
   margarine
1 glass milk

Lunch

Raspberry Purée (page 87)
Braised Cold Tongue with Aspic
   (page 89)

Mixed Vegetable Salad (page
   102)
Vanilla Yogurt
Perrier water (no ice)

Dinner

Rice Ring De Luxe (page 114)
Meat Loaf Special (page 91)
Applesauce Brûlée (page 104)

coffee (if permitted) with cream
and sugar

(IF THE DOCTOR LIMITS THE CONSUMPTION OF MILK OR MILK PRODUCTS)

Breakfast

Broiled Grapefruit (page 106)
¼ pound boiled chicken livers
(mashed with salt and
margarine)

2 slices white toast
tea (if permitted)

Lunch

Raspberry Purée (page 87)
Braised Cold Tongue with Aspic
(page 89)
Mixed Vegetable Salad   (page
102)

Grape Gelatin Special   (page
157)
Perrier water (no ice)

Dinner

Rice Ring De Luxe (page 114)
Meat Loaf Special (page 91)

Applesauce Brûlée (page 104)
black coffee (if permitted)

7

Breakfast

canned black cherries
Cream of Wheat with milk and
light brown sugar
1 poached egg on toasted

English muffin
Simple Hollandaise Dressing
(page 129)
tea (if permitted)

Lunch

Beef and Barley Soup (page 84)
Cranberry-Pineapple Salad
(page 101)

soda crackers
Aimee's Apple Whip (page 104)
ginger ale (no ice)

121

Dinner

Escalloped Chicken and Noodles
  (page 90)
Yale Beets (page 96)
Boiled Asparagus (page 94)

Prune Snow Pudding (page 105)
coffee (if permitted) with cream
  and sugar

(IF THE DOCTOR LIMITS THE CONSUMPTION OF MILK OR MILK PRODUCTS)

Breakfast

1 poached egg on toasted
  English muffin
Simple Hollandaise Dressing
  (page 129)

toasted English muffin (2nd)
  with guava jelly
tea (if permitted)

Lunch

Beef and Barley Soup
  (page 84)
Cranberry-Pineapple Salad
  (page 101)

soda crackers
Aimee's Apple Whip
  (page 104)
ginger ale (no ice)

Dinner

Escalloped Chicken and
  Noodles (page 90)
Yale Beets (page 96)

Boiled Asparagus (page 94)
Prune Snow Pudding (page 105)
black coffee (if permitted)

5. Bland Peptic-Ulcer and Low-Residue Diet Sauces, Dressings, Icings, and Frostings

The Bland Diet for Peptic Ulcer—any of the following recipes may be used.

The Bland Low-Residue Diet—any of the following recipes may be used except those containing milk or milk products if the doctor has limited the patient's consumption of such foods.

White Sauce

THIN WHITE SAUCE
1 tablespoon butter or margarine
1 tablespoon flour
¼ teaspoon salt
1 cup milk
Yield: 1 cup

MEDIUM WHITE SAUCE

2 tablespoons butter or margarine
2 tablespoons flour
Yield: 1 cup

¼ teaspoon salt
1 cup milk

THICK WHITE SAUCE

3 tablespoons butter or margarine
4 tablespoons flour
Yield: 1 cup

¼ teaspoon salt
1 cup milk

To prepare a Basic White Sauce: Melt the butter or margarine in a small saucepan over low heat. Blend in the flour and salt. Add the milk, stirring the mixture constantly until it thickens and bubbles.

The Thin White Sauce is very useful in making the cream of vegetable soups recommended for use during the early convalescence of the peptic-ulcer patient.

The Medium White Sauce is used as a base for sauces of various kinds and for creamed dishes.

The Thick White Sauce is used in making soufflés and croquettes.

Variations of the White Sauce

CHEESE SAUCE

2 to 4 ounces mild American cheese, grated
1 cup Medium or Thin White Sauce
Paprika (optional)

Set the mixture of cheese and sauce over hot water and stir until the cheese is thoroughly blended with the sauce. Season with a dash of paprika, if desired.
Yield: 1 cup

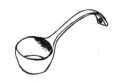

EGG SAUCE

Add one chopped, hard-boiled egg to one cup Medium White Sauce.

Yield: 1 cup

PARSLEY SAUCE

Add two to four tablespoons chopped parsley to one cup Medium or Thin White Sauce.

Yield: 1 cup

OYSTER SAUCE

Heat one pint of small oysters in their own liquor to boiling point. Boil one-half minute, and combine with one cup of Medium White Sauce.

Yield: 1 cup

Lemon Sauce

1 cup margarine   3 tablespoons lemon juice

Remove the margarine from the refrigerator one hour before preparing the sauce. Stir the lemon juice into the softened margarine. Blend the two ingredients thoroughly. This sauce is for immediate use. It adds zest to fish, meat, or vegetable dishes.

Yield: 1 cup

Lemon-Margarine Sauce

1½ tablespoons lemon juice   ¼ cup melted margarine

Beat the lemon juice into the margarine.

Yield: ¼ cup

Molasses Sauce

1 cup light molasses   1 tablespoon lemon juice
1½ tablespoons margarine

Boil the molasses with the margarine in a small saucepan over low heat for five minutes. Remove from the stove. Slowly stir in the lemon juice. This sauce is especially good on Brown Betty (page 156).

Yield: 1 cup

Special Tomato Sauce

2½ cups canned tomatoes	2 tablespoons margarine
½ teaspoon salt	2 tablespoons flour

Simmer the tomatoes with the salt briefly in a medium saucepan. Push through a sieve or food mill to remove the seeds. Melt the margarine in the original saucepan. Stir in the flour. Add the tomatoes gradually. Stir until the mixture boils and thickens. Cook for about three minutes longer, stirring occasionally. This sauce is especially good with timbales, meat loaves, or fish.

Yield: 2½ cups

Yogurt Sauce

1 cup unflavored yogurt	2 tablespoons finely
2 tablespoons lemon juice	chopped parsley
1 teaspoon salt	Dash of paprika

Combine all the ingredients. Mix thoroughly, but do not heat. Serve the sauce immediately.

Yield: 1 cup

Currant-Orange Sauce

1 cup currant jelly	½ cup orange juice

Break the jelly into small pieces with a fork. Add the orange juice. Let stand for one hour in the refrigerator before serving with chicken, lamb, or veal.

Yield: 1½ cups

Special Fish Sauce

¼ cup margarine	¼ cup minced cooked
½ teaspoon salt	shrimp

Cream the margarine until soft. Add the salt and the shrimp. Beat until fluffy. Spoon over fish just before serving.

Yield ½ cup

Crumb Sauce

½	cup melted margarine	1	teaspoon minced parsley
5	tablespoons dry white bread crumbs		Salt

Mix the margarine, crumbs, and parsley. Add salt to taste. Simmer until browned. Serve hot. Good with asparagus and stewed tomatoes.

Yield: ¾ cup

Apricot Dessert Sauce

3	tablespoons margarine	3	drops almond extract
1	cup sifted confectioners' sugar	4	tablespoons canned apricot nectar
1	tablespoon lemon juice		

Cream together the margarine and sugar. Add the lemon juice, almond extract, and apricot nectar. Beat until well blended. Serve cold over vanilla ice cream, plain boiled white rice, tapioca pudding, custard.

Yield: about 1¼ cups

Cooked Orange Dessert Sauce

½	cup sugar	½	cup boiling water
⅛	teaspoon salt	½	cup orange juice, heated
1	tablespoon cornstarch	2	tablespoons margarine

Mix the sugar, salt, and cornstarch in a small saucepan. Slowly stir in the water and orange juice. Cook over low heat, stirring, until the mixture thickens. Remove from the heat. Add the margarine. Serve warm over sliced pound cake, vanilla cornstarch, pudding, corn meal mush.

Yield: about ⅔ cup

Orange Sauce

| 1 | egg white | 3 | drops lemon extract |
| ¼ | cup confectioners' sugar | 5 | tablespoons orange juice |

Beat the egg white until stiff. Gradually add the sugar, lemon extract, and orange juice. Beat until well blended. Serve immediately. Good with beet salad, cold roast duck, cold sliced ham.

Yield: about ¾ cup

Vanilla Dessert Sauce

⅔	cup sugar	2	tablespoons margarine
1	tablespoon flour	1	teaspoon vanilla extract
1	cup boiling water		

Mix the sugar and flour together in a small saucepan. Gradually add the water. Cook, stirring constantly. When thickened, add the margarine. Remove from the heat. Add the vanilla extract.

Yield: 1 cup

Mock Whipped Cream Topping

½	cup dried milk powder	3	tablespoons sugar
½	cup ice water	½	teaspoon vanilla extract
1	tablespoon lemon juice		

Chill a medium mixing bowl and an eggbeater or a whisk for one hour. Pour the milk powder and water into the chilled bowl. Beat until the mixture is stiff enough to form peaks. Add the lemon juice slowly and continue beating for two minutes. Stir in the sugar and vanilla extract. Serve immediately as dessert topping. This topping must not be heated.

Yield: 1½ cups

Rum-Flavored Mock Whipped Cream Topping

½	cup dried milk powder	2	teaspoons sugar
½	cup ice water	¼	teaspoon rum extract
2	tablespoons lemon juice		

Chill a medium mixing bowl and an eggbeater or a whisk for one hour. Pour the milk powder and water into the chilled bowl. Beat until the mixture is stiff enough to form peaks. Add the lemon juice slowly and continue beating for two minutes. Stir in the sugar and rum extract. Serve immediately as dessert topping. Do not heat.

Yield: 1½ cups

Pink Lady Topping

1 egg white, unbeaten	⅓ cup grape jelly
	Pinch of salt

Combine the ingredients in the top of a double boiler. Beat with a rotary beater while cooking. When the mixture is stiff, remove from the stove. Cool. This topping cannot be reheated.

Yield: ½ cup

Fruit Juice Salad Dressing

2 eggs, lightly beaten	¼ cup lemon juice
¼ cup orange juice	½ cup sugar

Combine the ingredients in the top of a double boiler until thick.

Yield: 1 scant cup

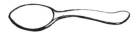

Simple Hollandaise Sauce

2 egg yolks	2 tablespoons margarine,
2 tablespoons lemon juice	melted
½ teaspoon salt	

Beat the egg yolks vigorously. Add the lemon juice, salt, and margarine. Whip the combined ingredients with a whisk. Cook in the top of a double boiler until thick, stirring constantly.

Yield: ¾ cup

Sour Cream Dressing

1 cup sour cream	2 tablespoons lemon juice
1 tablespoon honey	1 tablespoon sugar

Combine all the ingredients. Mix well. Chill until ready to use. This dressing should never be heated.

Yield: 1¼ cups

Cottage Cheese Dressing

1 cup cottage cheese	1½ cups sour cream
1 tablespoon sugar	¼ teaspoon salt
2 teaspoons lemon juice	

Combine all the ingredients in a large bowl. Mix them well, using a large spoon, whisk, or blender. Refrigerate. Serve somewhat chilled but not icy.

Yield: 2½ cups

Cream Cheese Icing

4 tablespoons margarine	2 cups sifted
1 three-ounce package	confectioners' sugar
cream cheese	1 teaspoon vanilla extract

Mix all the ingredients in a large bowl. Beat with an electric beater.

Yield: 2½ cups

Mamma's Special Icing

1½ cups confectioners' sugar	1 teaspoon vanilla extract
3 tablespoons milk	

Combine all the ingredients in a small bowl. Mix well until of spreading consistency.

Yield: about 1½ cups

130

Simple Sponge Cake Icing

1	egg white	3	tablespoons water
⅛	teaspoon cream of tartar	½	teaspoon lemon extract
½	cup sugar		

Combine the egg white, cream of tartar, sugar, and water in the top of a double boiler. Cook, beating constantly, until the mixture stands up in peaks. Remove from the heat. Add the lemon extract and beat well. This icing is good on angel food cake as well as on sponge cake.

Yield: ¾ cup

Boiled Cake Frosting

1½	cups sugar	2	egg whites
½	cup water	⅛	teaspoon salt
1	tablespoon light corn syrup	1	teaspoon vanilla extract

Combine the sugar, water, and corn syrup in a medium saucepan. Stir over low heat until the sugar is dissolved. Boil, covered, for about three minutes. Remove the cover. Boil, without stirring, until a small amount of the syrup forms a ball when dropped into cold water. Remove the syrup from the heat. Beat the egg whites in a medium bowl until stiff. Pour syrup in a fine stream over the egg whites, beating constantly. Add the salt and vanilla extract. Continue beating until the frosting is cool and spreadable.

Yield: frosting for top and sides of two nine-inch layers or two dozen cup cakes

Creamy Orange Frosting

½	cup soft margarine	2	teaspoons vanilla
3	tablespoons orange juice	3	cups confectioners' sugar

Mix all the ingredients in a large bowl. Beat until smooth.
Yield: 3½ cups

Simple Uncooked Frosting

1 egg white, unbeaten
½ cup light corn syrup

½ teaspoon vanilla extract
Dash of salt

Combine all the ingredients in a medium bowl. Beat until fluffy and spreadable. Refrigerate if not used within a few hours.
Yield: 1 cup

6. The Bland Low-Fat Diet

"Fair, fat, and forty" is the term frequently used to describe the female gallbladder patient. Unfeeling, but not inaccurate. The individual suffering from an ailing gall bladder is apt to be a woman, fortyish or more, who is no sylph, although that is not to say that a slender man of fifty (give or take a few years) may not have a gallbladder problem!

The two most common gallbladder complaints—inflammation of the organ (cholecystitis) or the presence of gallstones (cholethiasis)—often cause severe pain.

Fat in the diet is responsible for contraction of the diseased gallbladder and therefore for much of the pain entailed. A low-fat regime is a very important phase of the gallbladder patient's care. Bulky, highly spiced foods which can cause distress are also contraindicated.

Surgical removal of the gallbladder is frequently in order. When it is considered necessary, a weight-loss program before surgery may be inaugurated.

A major difference between the bland low-fat diet and the bland diet for peptic ulcer lies in food preparation which, in the former case, entails restriction of fats.

The list of "permitted" and "forbidden" foods given for a patient on the bland diet for peptic ulcer (page 28) is valid for the patient on the bland low-fat diet, with the exceptions noted below. Persons on the low-fat diet may use the recipes given for the bland diet for peptic ulcer and the bland low-residue diet by making the substitutions and omissions noted below. Those on the peptic ulcer and low-residue diets should consult their physicians before embarking on a low-fat regime.

133

Low-Fat Diet:

No whole milk. Skimmed milk must be substituted in milk drinks, sauces, soups, and desserts. Evaporated skimmed milk must be substituted for light cream.

Mildly seasoned meat-stock soups are permitted. They should be chilled after cooking and the fat skimmed off.

The physician should be consulted regarding the amount of butter or margarine, vegetable oils, and egg yolks that may be used with meals and in cooking.

Only lean meats and fish with a low-fat content are permitted.

Consult the doctor regarding the use of finely shredded raw lettuce and uncooked, skinned, seeded tomatoes.

Cottage cheese must be uncreamed. Cream cheese must be low-fat (called "imitation" cream cheese). Low-fat yogurt may be used.

Bananas are the only raw fruit permitted.

Angel food cake is the only type of cake permitted.

Coffee, tea, and decaffeinated coffee may be used if the doctor approves, but they are to be served without cream or whole milk.

No alcohol or carbonated beverages may be consumed.

Soups

Apricot and Apple Soup

2	cups strained apricot pulp	¾	cup sugar
2	cups strained apple pulp	4	tablespoons lemon juice
1	cup orange juice	¼	cup quick-cooking tapioca
½	teaspoon cinnamon		Pinch of salt

Place all the ingredients in the top of a double boiler. Simmer for fifteen minutes or until the tapioca is transparent and the soup hot.

Yield: 4 servings

Cold Asparagus Soup

1	pound fresh asparagus	1	teaspoon salt
1	tablespoon finely chopped parsley	2	cups skimmed milk
¼	teaspoon mace	½	cup evaporated skimmed milk

Wash the asparagus thoroughly. Snap off and discard the rough ends. Cut the tender portions in one-inch lengths. Combine with the parsley, mace, and salt. Cook in boiling, salted water until the asparagus is just tender (fifteen to twenty minutes). Drain. Combine with one cup of the skimmed milk in the blender container. Blend until smooth. Add the remaining skimmed milk. Blend for about ten seconds. Add the evaporated skimmed milk. Blend for another ten seconds. Chill. Serve in bouillon cups.

Yield: 6 servings

Cream of Oyster Soup

1	pint oysters	Salt
4	cups non-fat, reliquefied milk	Paprika
2	tablespoons quick-cooking tapioca	Oysterette crackers

Pick over the oysters. Remove any bits of shell. Cook the oysters in a small saucepan in their own liquor until their edges curl. Bring milk to a boil in a large saucepan. Add the tapioca. Stir constantly as the mixture thickens. Add the oysters and their liquor to the milk and tapioca mixture. Salt to taste. Serve hot. Sprinkle with paprika. Oysterette crackers go well with this soup.

Yield: 6 servings

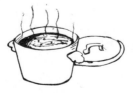

135

Hearty Old-Fashioned Soup

2 pounds lean beef, cut into one-inch cubes
2 pounds beef bones, cracked
2 quarts water
2 medium carrots, sliced crosswise
2 tablespoons salt
⅓ cup lemon juice
2 tablespoons sugar
   Allspice
2 sprigs parsley, finely chopped
4 slices day-old white bread, toasted

Cover the meat and bones with the water. Bring slowly to a boil. Skim. Add the carrots and salt. Cover the pot and simmer for one hour. Stir in the lemon juice, sugar, and a dash of allspice. Cover and simmer for one hour longer. Remove the bones. Refrigerate the soup overnight, or for several hours, so that the fat will rise to the surface where it can be skimmed off. When reheating to serve, add the parsley and cook for five minutes. Cut the toast into small cubes, and sprinkle a few cubes over each serving.

Yield: 8 servings

Tomato Bisque

4 cups skimmed milk
¾ cup zwieback crumbs
1 tablespoon finely chopped parsley
½ bay leaf
½ teaspoon thyme
2 cups canned tomatoes
2 teaspoons sugar
⅓ teaspoon baking soda
½ tablespoon salt
   Pilot crackers

Scald the milk with the crumbs, parsley, bay leaf, and thyme in a medium saucepan. Cook the tomatoes and sugar for fifteen minutes in a separate small saucepan. Add the baking soda. Push through a sieve to remove seeds. Remove the bay leaf from the milk-crumb mixture. Reheat to the boiling point. Add the tomatoes and salt. Reheat. Pour into a tureen. Serve with Pilot crackers.

Yield: 6 servings

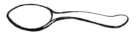

Turkey Bone Soup

Bones of one cooked turkey
½ teaspoon salt
2 quarts cold water
2 carrots, sliced crosswise
2 cups canned tomatoes
¼ bay leaf
¼ teaspoon thyme

¼ cup cooked white rice
Small bits of cooked
turkey meat (optional)
2 cups Chicken Broth
(page 86) (optional)
1 sprig parsley, finely
chopped

Place the turkey bones and salt in a large kettle with the water. Bring to a boil. Simmer gently, tightly covered, for two hours. Add the carrots, tomatoes, bay leaf, and thyme. Bring to a boil. Simmer for another half-hour. Cool. Remove the bones and the bay leaf. Add the rice. If desired, add bits of cooked turkey meat and the homemade chicken broth. When reheating the soup to serve, add the parsley and simmer for ten minutes.

Yield: 6 servings

Unbeatable Beet Soup

2 cups canned sliced beets
3 tablespoons sugar
2 tablespoons lemon juice
¼ teaspoon salt

¼ teaspoon allspice
2 cups water
1 cup cold evaporated
skimmed milk

Drain the beets. Reserve the liquid. Chop the beets finely and push through a food mill. In a medium saucepan combine the puréed beets, beet juice, sugar, lemon juice, salt, allspice, and water. Bring to a boil. Simmer for five minutes. Remove from the heat. Chill. Before serving, beat in the milk.

Yield: 4 to 5 servings

Vegetable Beef Soup

3 pounds beef shank
1 one-pint, two-ounce can
tomato juice
4 teaspoons salt
2 quarts water
1 one-pound can tomatoes
1 cup sliced carrots

1 cup diced potatoes
1 ten-ounce package
frozen lima beans
2 sprigs parsley, finely
chopped
2 bay leaves

Combine the meat, tomato juice, salt, and water in a large soup kettle. Cover and simmer gently for two hours. Cool. Cut the meat from the bones in large cubes. Strain the broth. Refrigerate until the fat rises to the top and can be skimmed off. Return the meat and the broth to the soup kettle. Add the remaining ingredients. Cover and simmer for one hour.

Yield: 8 servings

Meats

Baked Chicken Delight

1 three-pound frying chicken, cut in serving pieces	2 tablespoons finely chopped parsley
2 cups evaporated skimmed milk	1 teaspoon salt
	1 teaspoon allspice
	2 cups zwieback crumbs

Remove the skin and dip the chicken pieces into the milk. Combine the parsley, salt, and allspice. Sprinkle over the chicken. Roll each piece in the crumbs. Arrange in a medium baking pan which has been lined with aluminum foil. Cover the chicken pieces completely with foil. Bake at 350 degrees for about one hour, or until fork-tender.

Yield: 4 servings

Barbecued Chicken à la Back Yard

2 tablespoons lemon juice	¼ teaspoon allspice
1 cup tomato juice	1 two-and-a-half- to three-pound frying chicken, cut in quarters
1 teaspoon salt	
1 teaspoon paprika	

Combine the first five ingredients for marinade. Marinate the chicken for two hours. Barbecue over charcoal on an outdoor grill or broil in the oven for fifteen minutes on each side. Baste with the marinade several times while cooking. Remove the skin before serving.

Yield: 4 servings

Broiled Lamb Chops

2 single lamb chops (loin, rib, or shoulder)	Mint jelly

Select chops of uniform thickness. Trim away any excess fat. Place on the broiling pan rack in preheated broiler. Turn when first side is brown, using kitchen tongs which do not pierce the meat. Broil according to whether you want the chops pink or well done. Serve with the jelly.

Yield: 1 or 2 servings

Cape Cod Pot Roast

4 pounds beef chuck or round	¼ cup water
2 cups canned jellied cranberry sauce	2 teaspoons salt
	¼ teaspoon cinnamon

If the beef is not in a solid piece, skewer or tie it into shape. Sear the meat in a Dutch oven, using a sprinkle of salt instead of grease. When the meat is browned on all sides, add the remaining ingredients. Cook slowly, tightly covered, for about three hours, or until the meat is tender. Turn frequently. Add additional water as necessary. When the meat is cooked, refrigerate, so any fat can be scraped off the meat and skimmed from any remaining gravy. Reheat to serve.

Yield: 6 to 8 servings

Chicken Little, Baked

1 two-and-a-half- to three-pound roasting chicken	¼ teaspoon finely chopped parsley
¼ teaspoon salt	¼ teaspoon thyme

Preheat the oven to 350 degrees. Combine the salt, parsley, and thyme. Sprinkle the inside of the chicken with these seasonings. Truss the legs and the wings to the body. Cover completely with aluminum foil. Place in the oven in a shallow medium baking pan. After 45 minutes, remove the foil. Raise the oven temperature to 450 degrees. Continue baking about twenty-five minutes, or until the chicken is golden brown. Remove the skin before serving.

Yield: 4 servings

Individual Meat Loaves

½	pound ground lean beef	1	four-ounce can sliced mushrooms (packed without butter)
½	pound ground lean lamb		
1	cup soft white bread crumbs	¼	teaspoon salt
2	egg whites	½	teaspoon allspice
¼	cup evaporated skimmed milk		Low-Fat Tomato Sauce (page 165)
1	tablespoon minced parsley		

Combine all the ingredients except the sauce. Mix well. Spoon into six custard cups or a six-cup muffin tin. Bake at 350 degrees for thirty minutes, or until done. Turn out the individual loaves. Top with the sauce before serving.

Yield: 6 servings

Jelly-Glazed Roast Lamb

1	five- to eight-pound leg of lamb		Salt
2	sprigs parsley, finely chopped	½	cup grape jelly
		½	cup hot water

Rub the lamb with the parsley. Sprinkle lightly with salt. Roast in a large roasting pan, uncovered, at 350 degrees. Allow twenty to thirty-five minutes per pound for medium-done meat, thirty to thirty-five minutes for well done. During the last hour of roasting, baste frequently with the jelly dissolved in the water. Serve on a hot platter.

Yield: 6 to 8 servings

London Broil à la John

2 pounds flank or round
  steak

Juice of 2 lemons
Salt

Marinate the meat in the lemon juice overnight in the refrigerator. Turn several times during the following morning. Remove from the marinade one hour before cooking. Preheat the broiler. Broil meat to desired degree of doneness, turning once. When well browned on both sides, sprinkle lightly with salt. The carving is as important as the cooking. A sharp knife and a carving board are imperative. Slice on the bias, across the grain of the meat, at a forty-five degree angle. Slices should be about one-quarter inch thick.

Yield: 4 to 5 servings

Maple-Glazed Lamb Steaks

½ cup maple syrup
¼ cup light brown sugar
3 tablespoons pineapple
  juice
1 tablespoon orange juice
2 sprigs fresh parsley,
  finely chopped

¼ teaspoon salt
2 lamb steaks, one-half
  inch thick, cut from a leg
  of lamb

Combine the first six ingredients in a small saucepan. Cook over low heat, stirring constantly. Place the lamb steaks on a rack in a roasting pan. Brush with the maple glaze. Roast at 350 degrees for about forty-five minutes. Baste frequently.

Yield: 2 servings

Plain Broiled Chicken

1 two-pound to
  two-and-a-half-pound
  broiling chicken

Lemon juice
Salt

Ask the butcher to quarter the chicken and break the wing and leg joints to flatten the chicken for broiling. Drizzle lemon juice over the chicken about four hours before serving time. Refrigerate. Bring to room temperature before cooking. Place, skin down, on a cookie sheet lined with aluminum foil. Brush generously with lemon juice. Sprinkle lightly with salt. Broil about six inches from the source of heat. Turn, after fifteen or twenty minutes, using kitchen tongs to avoid piercing the meat and thus causing a loss of juice. Brush, after turning, with lemon juice. Broil about twenty minutes longer. Watch the chicken constantly while broiling. Remove the skin before serving.

Yield: 4 servings

"Skinny" Parsley Meatballs

½	cup day-old white bread crumbs	¼	teaspoon allspice
¼	cup skimmed milk	¼	cup finely chopped parsley
1	pound lean ground beef		Low-Fat Tomato Sauce
2	egg whites		(page 165)
1	teaspoon salt		

Soften the crumbs in the milk. Mix together with the next five ingredients. Form into 6 meatballs. Panbroil in large iron skillet (see page 41). Top with sauce before serving.

Yield: 3 to 6 servings

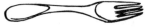

"Skinny" Pineapple Meat Loaf

1¼	pounds lean ground beef	¼	teaspoon thyme
1	eight-ounce can crushed pineapple with natural unsweetened juice	¼	teaspoon mace
2	slices white bread, cubed	1	tablespoon minced parsley
2	egg whites		Low-Fat Tomato Sauce
½	teaspoon salt		(page 165)

Mix together all the ingredients except the sauce. Form into a loaf. Bake for one hour and fifteen minutes at 350 degrees in a nine-inch loaf pan. Cut into six slices. When serving, top with the sauce.

Yield: 6 servings

Turkey Casserole

1 four-ounce can sliced
  mushrooms, packed
  without butter
  Skimmed milk
2 tablespoons
  quick-cooking tapioca
½ teaspoon salt
1½ cups cooked white rice

2 cups diced, cooked
  turkey
1 ten-ounce package
  frozen cut asparagus,
  thawed
½ cup dry white bread
  crumbs

Preheat the oven to 375 degrees. Drain the mushrooms, reserving the liquid. Add enough milk to the mushroom liquid to measure two cups. Heat in a medium saucepan. Add the tapioca and salt. Boil the mixture for about five minutes, stirring as it thickens. Remove from the heat. Stir the mushrooms into the sauce. In an ungreased, medium, deep casserole, layer half of the rice, half of the turkey, and half of the asparagus. Pour half of the mushroom sauce over the top. Repeat the layers, finishing with the remaining sauce. Sprinkle with the crumbs. Bake, uncovered, for 35 minutes, or until the crumbs are brown.

Yield: 6 to 8 servings

Vegetables

Baked Acorn Squash (Low-Fat Version)

Refer to the Baked Acorn Squash Recipe (page 50), but make the following changes. Turn the squash halves cut side up. Omit the margarine, and use

1 tablespoon honey
2 teaspoons orange juice

Cinnamon

Combine the honey and orange juice. Pour into the squash cavities. Add a sprinkle of cinnamon. Bake for another twenty minutes or until the squash is soft.

Yield: 2 to 4 servings

Asparagus Treat

Boiled Asparagus (page 94)

1 cup Low-Fat Yogurt Sauce (page 165)

Cook the asparagus according to the recipe, but use the Low-Fat Yogurt Sauce instead of the Simple Hollandaise Sauce. Serve cold.

Yield: 4 servings

Baked Carrots

6 medium carrots
1 cup water
½ cup honey

¼ teaspoon salt
½ teaspoon allspice

Wash and scrape the carrots. Cut in julienne strips. Place in a small baking dish. Add the water and honey. Sprinkle with the salt and allspice. Bake, covered, for about forty-five minutes at 400 degrees. Remove the cover to brown.

Yield: 3 servings

Green Beans and Mushrooms

1 sixteen-ounce can cut green beans
2 tablespoons cornstarch
1 cup skimmed milk
¼ teaspoon salt
1 four-ounce can sliced mushrooms (packed without butter), drained

1 tablespoon finely chopped parsley
¼ teaspoon mace

Drain the beans, reserving the liquid. In a medium saucepan, blend the cornstarch well with ¼ cup of the green bean liquid. Cook, stirring constantly, while gradually adding the milk and salt. When the sauce has thickened, stir in the green beans, mushrooms, parsley, and mace. Mix well. Heat and serve.

Yield: 6 servings

Marmalade Beets

2 cups canned beets	¼ cup marmalade, strained
¼ teaspoon allspice	4 tablespoons orange juice

Drain the beets. Chop finely. Combine with the remaining ingredients. Cook over low heat, stirring constantly, for about ten minutes, until the beets are hot.

Yield: 4 servings

Mashed Carrots

6 medium carrots	¼ teaspoon salt
¼ cup evaporated skimmed milk	Dash of mace
	1 teaspoon honey

Halve the carrots crosswise. Steam, covered, over boiling water. When soft, rinse in cold water. Skin the carrot halves, cut them into thin slices, and place them in a large mixing bowl. Mash. Add the remaining ingredients. Beat vigorously until light and fluffy. Heat in the top of a double boiler before serving.

Yield: 3 servings

Maple Sweet Potatoes

6 medium sweet potatoes	½ cup skimmed milk
½ teaspoon salt	2 tablespoons maple syrup
Allspice	

Boil, peel, and mash the sweet potatoes. Add the salt, a dash of allspice, and the milk. Whisk until light and fluffy. Turn into a greased medium baking dish. Top with the maple syrup. Bake at 350 degrees for about twenty-five minutes.

Yield: 6 servings

Newport Spinach

1 pound spinach	½ teaspoon salt
2 sprigs parsley	Cinnamon
3 tablespoons flour	¼ cup evaporated skimmed milk
2 cups skimmed milk	

145

Wash the spinach and the parsley. Cut out the stems. Cook. Chop very fine. Mix the flour with a little cold water to make a paste. Gradually add the skimmed milk. Simmer until thick and smooth, stirring constantly. Add the spinach and parsley. Season with the salt and a dash of cinnamon. Pour in the evaporated milk. Stir, heat, and serve.

Yield: 3 servings

Parsleyed Asparagus

7   asparagus tips (fresh or frozen)
Salt
1   tablespoon finely chopped parsley

1   slice hot unbuttered toast
Mace

As the asparagus tips are cooking, add a pinch of salt and the parsley. When tender, serve hot on the hot toast. Top with a dash of mace.

Yield: 1 serving

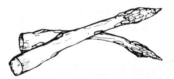

Pineapple Acorn Squash

3   medium acorn squash
1   eight and three-quarter-ounce can crushed pineapple

1¼   cups chopped apple
2   tablespoons light brown sugar

Halve the squash crosswise. Remove the seeds and the stringy fibers. Drain the pineapple. (Reserve the liquid for future use in a beverage.) Combine the pineapple, apple, and sugar. Place the squash cut side up in a small, shallow baking pan. Fill the cavities with the fruit and sugar mixture. Cover with aluminum foil. Bake for one hour at 350 degrees. Test for doneness. If not fork-tender, bake a bit longer.

Yield: 6 servings

Succotash

1½ cups canned cream-style corn
1½ cups canned lima beans
Sprinkle of salt

¼ teaspoon mace
½ cup evaporated skimmed milk

Turn the corn into a medium saucepan. Drain the lima beans and discard the liquid. Add the beans to the corn. Add the remaining ingredients. Heat and serve.

Yield: 6 servings

Fish and Shellfish

Baked Haddock

2 pounds haddock steak (or other non-fatty fish steak)
Lemon juice
½ teaspoon salt

1½ cups evaporated skimmed milk
Paprika

Brush the fish generously with lemon juice. Let stand one hour before cooking. Place in a medium baking dish. Salt lightly. Pour the milk over the fish. Bake at 350 degrees for forty-five minutes, basting frequently. Sprinkle with paprika before serving.

Yield: 4 servings

Cod Fillets with Mushroom Sauce

1 pound frozen cod fillets
Lemon juice
1 cup skimmed milk
¼ teaspoon salt
2 tablespoons flour

1 four-ounce can sliced mushrooms (packed without butter), drained
1 sprig parsley, finely chopped
Paprika

Allow the fillets to thaw at room temperature. Brush generously with lemon juice. Arrange in a shallow baking dish. Set aside. Blend the milk and salt with the flour. Cook over medium heat, stirring constantly, until the sauce becomes thick and bubbly. Add the mushrooms and parsley. Cook for another five minutes. Pour the sauce over the fish. Bake, uncovered, at 350 degrees, for about 25 minutes. Dust lightly with paprika before serving.

Yield: 4 servings

Leftover Fish and Cottage Cheese Mold

2 envelopes unflavored gelatin	1 cup uncreamed cottage cheese
2 cups clam juice	Paprika
1 teaspoon salt	
1 tablespoon lemon juice	
1 pound leftover cooked haddock or other non-fatty fish	

Sprinkle the gelatin over one cup of the clam juice in a medium saucepan. Stir constantly over low heat for about three minutes until the gelatin dissolves. Remove from the heat. Stir in the remaining cup of clam juice, the salt, and lemon juice. Chill, stirring occasionally, until the mixture is slightly thicker than unbeaten egg white in consistency. Pick over the fish, removing any skin and bones. Flake with a fork. Fold, with the cheese, into the gelatin mixture. Turn into a five-cup mold. Chill until firm. Unmold. Dust with paprika before serving.

Yield: 5 servings

Poached Fish with Yogurt Sauce

2 pounds fresh fish (cod, halibut, whitefish, or pike)	2 tablespoons lemon juice
	2 sprigs parsley, finely chopped
1 bay leaf	Low-Fat Yogurt Sauce (page 165)
½ teaspoon allspice	

Envelop the fish in a piece of cheesecloth. Place in a medium saucepan, in just enough boiling water to cover. Add the bay leaf, allspice, lemon juice, and parsley. Cover lightly. Simmer the fish gently for about fifteen minutes. Test with a fork for flaking, which indicates doneness. Chill when cooked. Serve cold with the sauce.

Yield: 4 to 5 servings

Baked Oysters with Spinach

1 ten-ounce package frozen chopped spinach	½ cup Chicken Broth (page 86)
1 pint oysters	¼ cup water
Evaporated skimmed milk	1 tablespoon cornstarch
	Paprika

Cook the spinach according to the package directions. Pick over the oysters. Remove any bits of shell. Drain the oyster liquor into a measuring cup. Add enough milk to equal 1 cup. Add the chicken broth. Set aside. Mix the water with the cornstarch in a medium saucepan. Cook, stirring constantly. Add the oyster liquor, milk, and broth mixture. Cook, stirring, until the sauce boils and thickens. Remove from the heat. Spread the spinach in the bottom of a medium casserole. Spoon the oysters over the spinach. Pour the sauce over the oysters. Dust lightly with paprika. Bake at 375 degrees for about twenty minutes.

Yield: 5 servings

Panned Oysters

1 pint large oysters	Paprika
¼ cup oyster liquor	Lemon wedges
6 slices white bread, toasted	

Preheat the oven to 450 degrees. Pick over the oysters. Remove any bits of shell. Drain. Arrange the oysters in a small shallow baking pan. Pour the oyster liquor over them. Place the pan in the oven and leave it just long enough for the oysters to heat through. Moisten the toast with the hot oyster liquor. Serve the oysters on the toast. Add a dash of paprika to each serving, and place a lemon wedge on the side.

Yield: 3 servings

Scalloped Oysters

1 cup soft white bread crumbs	¼ teaspoon mace
1 cup ground zwieback crumbs	2 tablespoons finely chopped parsley
1 pint oysters, drained (reserve the liquor)	½ cup evaporated skimmed milk
¼ teaspoon salt	½ cup oyster liquor

Mix the bread crumbs and the zwieback crumbs. Pick over the oysters. Remove any bits of shell. In a medium baking dish arrange a layer of one-third of the crumbs, then a layer of half of the oysters. Sprinkle lightly with salt, mace, parsley. Repeat the layering procedure and sprinkle again with the seasonings. Top with the remaining crumbs. Mix together the milk and oyster liquor. Moisten the contents of the baking dish with this combination. Bake at 350 degrees about thirty minutes, or until the top is brown.

Yield: 6 servings

Oysters Baked in the Shell

7 medium oysters	Salt
Lemon juice	Allspice

Preheat the oven to 500 degrees. Wash the oyster shells well, using a brush. Arrange the oysters in a baking pan with the deep shell down. Place in the oven. Bake until the shells open. Add a squirt of lemon juice, a light sprinkling of salt, and a dash of allspice. Serve immediately.

Yield: 1 serving

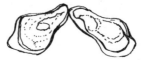

Salads

Applesauce Delight (Low-Fat Version)

Follow the Low-Residue Diet version of this recipe (page 100), but substitute Pink Lady Topping (page 129) for the Fruit Juice Salad Dressing.

Yield: 4 servings

Cold Asparagus Salad (Low-Fat Version)

8 canned asparagus tips	Low-Fat Cottage Cheese
Shredded lettuce leaf	Dressing (page 164)

Arrange the asparagus tips on very finely shredded lettuce leaf. (Eat the lettuce only with the doctor's permission.) Top with the dressing.

Yield: 1 serving

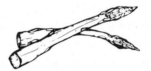

Mixed Fruit Salad (Low-Fat Version)

1 three-ounce package cherry-flavored gelatin	1 cup canned crushed pineapple, drained
1 cup boiling water	Rum-Flavored Mock
1 cup cold water	Whipped Cream Topping
1 cup canned peach slices, drained	(page 128)

Dissolve the gelatin in the boiling water. Add the cold water. Set aside to cool. Add the fruit. Pour into a mold which has been rinsed with cold water. Unmold when the gelatin has set. Add the topping when ready to serve.

Yield: 4 servings

Molded Cranberry Salad

1 three-ounce package
  strawberry-flavored
  gelatin
1 cup boiling water
1 cup cranberry juice
1 sixteen-ounce can jellied
  cranberry sauce

Finely shredded lettuce
leaves (to be eaten only
with doctor's
permission)
Low-Fat Cottage Cheese
Topping (page 164)

Dissolve the gelatin in the water. Add the cranberry juice. Chill until the gelatin begins to thicken. Fold in the cranberry sauce. Pour into a six-cup mold that has been rinsed in cold water. Refrigerate until set. Unmold. Serve on a bed of the finely shredded lettuce leaves. Add the topping.

Yield: 5 servings

Peach Salad

Finely shredded lettuce
leaf (to be eaten only
with doctor's
permission)
1 cup uncreamed cottage
  cheese, drained
2 canned peach halves,
  drained (reserve the
  liquid)

2 stewed pitted prunes
2 tablespoons evaporated
  skimmed milk
2 teaspoons maraschino
  cherry juice

Arrange the lettuce on a salad plate. Mound the cheese on the lettuce. Place the peach halves, cut side up, on the cheese. Set a prune in each peach center. Mix the milk and cherry juice with 2 tablespoons of the reserved peach liquid. Pour over the salad.

Yield: 1 serving

Peachy Yogurt Salad

1 sixteen-ounce can peach
  halves

2 eight-ounce cartons
  peach-flavored low-fat
  yogurt

Drain the peaches. (Reserve the liquid for another occasion.) Spoon the peaches into 4 dessert dishes. Top with the yogurt. Serve at once.

Yield: 4 servings

Pear and Cheese Salad (Low-Fat Version)

Follow the Low-Residue Version of this recipe (page 103), substituting the "imitation" or low-fat cream cheese for the regular cheese.

Yield: 4 servings

Salade Julienne

1 cup canned julienne beets	leaves (only with the doctor's permission)
1 cup fresh green beans	Low-Fat Yogurt Sauce
Finely shredded lettuce	(page 165)

Place the beets in a strainer to drain thoroughly. Wash the green beans and cut them in long, matchlike strips. Steam, covered, over boiling water, until tender. Make nests of the shredded lettuce on four salad plates. Spoon the beans into the four nests. Mound the beets on the center of the green beans. Top each salad with ¼ cup of the sauce.

Yield: 4 servings

Tomato-Vegetable Salad

1 ten-ounce package frozen mixed vegetables	2 teaspoons sugar
1 envelope unflavored gelatin	¼ teaspoon salt
½ cup cold water	Dash of paprika
1½ cups tomato juice	Low-Fat Yogurt Sauce (page 165)

Cook the vegetables according to the package directions. Measure 1 cup to be used in this recipe. (Reserve the remainder for use in soup.) Sprinkle the gelatin over the water, in a medium bowl. Allow it to stand for five minutes. Heat the tomato juice with the next three ingredients just to the boiling point. Add to the gelatin and water. Stir until the gelatin is entirely dissolved. Chill. When it begins to thicken, add the cooked vegetables. Pour into four sherbet glasses. Chill until firm. Top with the sauce.

Yield: 4 servings

Yummy Raspberry Treat (Low-Fat Version)

Follow the Low-Residue Version of this recipe (page 104), substituting Low-Fat Yogurt Sauce (page 165) as topping.

Yield: 4 servings

Desserts

Apple-Apricot Bake

6 large baking apples	¼ teaspoon cinnamon
1 cup apricot nectar	1 tablespoon honey
1 cup evaporated skimmed milk	Apricot jam

Peel, core, and slice the apples. Arrange in a shallow baking dish. Combine the next four ingredients. Pour over the apple slices. Bake, covered, at 350 degrees for about 35 minutes, or until the apples are fork-tender. Top each with jam before serving.

Yield: 6 to 8 servings

Apple Whisk

4 tart apples	¼ teaspoon cream of tartar
½ cup honey	3 egg whites
1 tablespoon orange juice	Plum jelly
¼ teaspoon cinnamon	

Cut the apples into small pieces. Steam, covered, over boiling water. When soft, push through a food mill or a strainer. Add the honey, orange juice, and cinnamon. Add the cream of tartar to the egg whites. Whisk until stiff. Fold into the apple mixture. Spoon into sherbet glasses. Chill. Top with the jelly before serving.

Yield: 5 servings

Baked Canned Fruits

1 cup canned peach halves	2 tablespoons light brown
1 cup canned pear halves	sugar
2 tablespoons orange juice	Sprinkle of mace
2 teaspoons lemon juice	

Drain the canned fruit, reserving the liquid. Arrange fruit, cavity side up, in a large, shallow baking dish. Blend together the remaining ingredients. Brush the fruits with this combination. Pour one-half cup of the fruit liquid into the baking dish around the fruit. Bake at 400 degrees for about fifteen minutes until the fruit is heated through.

Yield: 4 servings

Baked "Skinny" Apples

6 large red apples	¼ teaspoon cinnamon
2 cups banana slices	6 large, cooked pitted
1 cup guava jelly	prunes
¼ cup honey	

Cut off the stem end of the apples. Remove the core. Scoop out pulp around the center, making a cup about three-quarter inch thick. Mash the banana. Combine with the jelly, honey, and cinnamon. Stuff the apples with this mixture. Bake, uncovered, at 375 degrees until the apples are fork-tender. Top each apple with a prune when serving. Do not eat the apple peel.

Yield: 6 servings

Baked Stuffed Apples

6 large red apples	½ cup dark brown sugar
1 cup banana slices	¼ teaspoon mace
1 cup currant jelly	Marshmallow Whip

Cut off the stem end of the apples. Remove the core. Scoop out part of the pulp, making a cup about three-quarter inch thick. Mash the banana. Combine the banana, jelly, brown sugar, and mace. Fill the apple cavities with this mixture. Bake, uncovered, at 375 degrees until tender. Top each apple when cool with a teaspoonful of the whip. Do not eat the apple peel.

Yield: 6 servings

Banana and Cranberry Bake

3 bananas	Mock Whipped Cream
2 tablespoons lime juice	Topping (page 128)
Cinnamon	
1 can jellied cranberry sauce	

Peel the bananas. Slice in half lengthwise. Brush with the lime juice. Arrange in a shallow medium baking dish which has been coated with non-caloric, no-fat cooking spray. Sprinkle with cinnamon. Spoon the cranberry sauce over the bananas. Bake at 375 degrees for about twenty minutes, or until the bananas are tender. Top with the Mock Whipped Cream.

Yield: 3 servings

Brown Betty

1 cup dry white bread crumbs	1 apple, peeled, cored, and sliced in rings
3½ cups peeled chopped apples	Rum-Flavored Mock Whipped Cream Topping (page 128)
½ cup honey	
1 cup water	

Mix all but two tablespoons of the crumbs with chopped apples. Place in a deep baking dish. Bring the honey and water to a boil. Pour over the apple and crumb mixture. Sprinkle the remaining crumbs on the top. Arrange the apple rings around the edge. Cover. Bake at 300 degrees for thirty minutes. Remove the cover. Bake for another forty-five minutes. Add the topping before serving.

Yield: 5 to 6 servings

Delectable Apricot Whip

1½ cups stewed apricots, strained	¼ teaspoon salt
	2 tablespoons sugar
¼ cup orange marmalade, strained	2 egg whites
	Lemon Icing (page 165)
1 tablespoon lemon juice	

Combine the first four ingredients. Whip the sugar into the egg whites until stiff. Fold into the apricot mixture. Serve in dessert dishes. Top with the icing.

Yield: 4 servings

Farina Delight

1 serving farina	1 teaspoon light brown sugar
¼ cup crushed pineapple in unsweetened juice	Mamma's Special Icing (page 130)
¼ teaspoon cinnamon	

Cook the farina according to the package directions. Immediately stir in the next three ingredients. Chill. Top with the icing.

Yield: 1 serving

Grape Gelatin Special

1 envelope unflavored gelatin	¼ cup orange juice
¼ cup cold water	¼ teaspoon cream of tartar
1 cup hot grape juice	3 egg whites
⅓ cup sugar	Pink Lady Topping (page 129)

Soak the gelatin in the water. Dissolve in the grape juice. Add the sugar and orange juice. Cool. Stir occasionally. When gelatin begins to thicken, whisk until frothy. Add the cream of tartar to the egg whites. Beat until peaks form. Fold into the gelatin-grape juice mixture. Beat until stiff. Spoon into sherbet glasses. Chill. Add the topping before serving.

Yield: 4 servings

Hot Peach Dessert

1	sixteen-ounce can peach halves	¼	teaspoon mace
2	tablespoons orange juice		Angel Food Cake (page 160)
2	tablespoons light brown sugar		

Drain the peaches, reserving the liquid. Arrange, cavity side up, in a large, shallow baking dish. Combine the orange juice, sugar, and mace. Drizzle over the peaches. Pour one-half cup of the peach liquid into the baking dish around the fruit. Bake at 400 degrees for about fifteen minutes, or until the fruit is heated through. Serve with modest portions of the cake.

Yield: 4 servings

Meringued Cherries

1	one-pound four-ounce can pitted sour red cherries	2½	tablespoons quick-cooking tapioca
¾	cup sugar	2	egg whites
	Salt	¼	teaspoon cream of tartar
¼	teaspoon almond extract	¼	cup sugar

Drain the cherries, reserving one-half cup of the liquid. Chop the cherries. Add the cherry liquid, one-half cup of the sugar, and a pinch of salt, almond extract, and tapioca. Cook, stirring constantly, until thickened. Beat the egg whites and the cream of tartar together until soft peaks form. Gradually add the remaining sugar. Beat until stiff. Pour the cherry mixture into a shallow, square baking dish. Top with mounds of the beaten egg whites. Bake at 300 degrees for about eight to ten minutes, or until the meringue is lightly browned. Cool for one hour at room temperature. Chill for two hours before serving.

Yield: 6 servings

New England Apricot Pudding

½ pound dried apricots
½ cup sugar
6 slices cinnamon toast
    (prepared without butter)

1 cup Simple Uncooked
    Frosting (page 132)

Soak the apricots overnight. Stew in water to cover until tender. Add the sugar. Arrange squares of the toast in the bottom and around the sides of a medium pudding dish. Pour in the boiling hot apricots. Cover the dish so that no steam can escape. Cool gradually, then chill. Cover the top with the frosting.

Yield: 6 servings

Orange-Tapioca Dessert

¼ cup quick-cooking
    tapioca
2½ cups orange juice
    Salt

½ cup sugar
    Mock Whipped Cream
    (page 128)

Combine the tapioca, orange juice, a dash of salt, and the sugar in a medium saucepan. Allow these to stand for five minutes. Bring to a boil over medium heat, stirring frequently. Cool for twenty minutes. Stir well. Serve in sherbet glasses. Top with a dollop of the cream.

Yield: 4 servings

Peachy Cheese Treat

⅓ cup skimmed milk
½ teaspoon vanilla extract
2 tablespoons honey
1 eight-ounce container
    uncreamed cottage
    cheese

3 cups canned peach
    halves
    Grape jelly

Combine the first four ingredients in a large bowl. Blend into a smooth sauce, using a rotary beater. Drain the peaches, reserving the liquid for another use. Cover with the sauce. Refrigerate. Before serving, top with six mounds of the jelly.

Yield: 6 servings

Angel Food Cake*

6	egg whites		Salt
¼	teaspoon cream of tartar	½	teaspoon vanilla extract
¾	cup sugar	½	cup cake flour

Beat the egg whites until foamy. Add the cream of tartar. Continue beating until stiff. Fold in half the sugar, a pinch of salt, and vanilla. Add the remaining sugar to the flour. Sift four times. Add gradually to the egg whites. Fold in gently until well blended. Pour into an ungreased tube pan. Bake at 350 degrees for forty to sixty minutes. Leave the cake in the pan to cool. Turn a large funnel upside down, set the inverted cake pan over the upturned end. Or set the pan on the neck of an empty ginger ale bottle while the cake cools.

Yield: 8 to 10 servings

*Note: Angel Food Cake is the only cake permitted on the bland low-fat diet.

One-Dish Specialties

Asparagus Luncheon Treat

Boiled Asparagus (page 94)

2 cups Steamed White Rice (page 164)

1 cup Low-Fat Yogurt Sauce (page 165)

Boil the asparagus according to the recipe. Serve on a bed of rice instead of toast. Top with the Low-Fat Yogurt Sauce in place of the Simple Hollandaise Sauce.

Yield: 4 servings

Carrot and Macaroni Luncheon

Baked Carrots (page 144)	Low-Fat Cottage Cheese
4 ounces macaroni	Dressing (page 164)

Prepare the carrots according to the recipe. Cook the macaroni according to the package directions. Arrange a serving of the macaroni in the middle of each of three luncheon plates. Spoon a serving of baked carrots on the macaroni. Top the carrots with the dressing.

Yield: 3 servings

Carrot-Spinach Surprise Luncheon

1 ten-ounce package frozen chopped spinach	Carrot Surprise (page 94)

Cook the spinach according to the package directions. Prepare the Carrot Surprise according to the recipe. Mound spinach in the center of four large serving plates. Top with the carrots and their sauce. Serve hot.

Yield: 4 servings

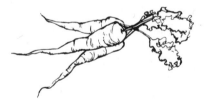

Green Bean and Mushroom Luncheon

Green Beans and Mushrooms (page 144)	Steamed White Rice (page 164)

Prepare the green beans and mushrooms according to the recipe. Cook the rice in a double boiler, following the recipe. Serve the hot vegetables and sauce over the steamed rice.

Yield: 6 servings

Macaroni and Tomato Luncheon

1 eight-ounce package macaroni Stewed Tomatoes (page 95)	2 tablespoons finely chopped parsley

Cook the macaroni according to the package directions. Prepare the tomatoes according to the recipe, but add the parsley. Combine the macaroni and tomatoes, mixing well with a large wooden spoon. Serve hot.

Yield: 6 servings

Mushrooms and Parsleyed Rice

2 four-ounce cans sliced mushrooms, packed without butter 3 tablespoons finely chopped parsley	1 tablespoon lemon juice 3 cups cooked white rice Paprika

Add the first three ingredients to the rice. Mix with a fork. Heat in the top of a double boiler. Mound on individual serving plates. Dust lightly with paprika.

Yield: 6 servings

Pineapple-Squash with Sweet Potato

1 medium acorn squash, cooked as in Pineapple Acorn Squash (page 146)	1 sweet potato Skimmed milk Salt

While preparing the acorn squash according to the recipe, wash the sweet potato and cut it in half. Cook, covered, in a small amount of boiling water for about thirty-five minutes, or until fork-tender. Peel after boiling. Mash the potato, using a small amount of skimmed milk and salt. Mound half the potato in the center of each of two luncheon plates. Scoop out the cooked center of the squash from the skin. Spoon half of the squash on top of each mound of sweet potato.

Yield: 2 servings

Potato and Pea Luncheon

1 baked potato	3 tablespoons canned
Dash of salt	green peas, heated and
3 tablespoons uncreamed	drained
cottage cheese	6 stewed pitted prunes,
	heated

Cut the potato and scoop out the pulp. Salt. Mash thoroughly. Fold in the cheese. Mound the potato and cheese mixture in the center of a luncheon plate. Top with the green peas. Arrange the prunes in a circle around the potato.

Yield: 1 serving

Rice Carioca

1 cup white rice	1 teaspoon salt
3 medium carrots, chopped	½ teaspoon allspice
1 pound lean ground beef	3 medium potatoes, peeled
1 teaspoon chopped	and diced
parsley	1 sixteen-ounce can
2 cups water	tomatoes

Wash and drain the rice. Combine with the next six ingredients. Mix lightly with a fork. Cook, covered, over low heat for fifteen minutes. Add the potatoes and tomatoes. Cook for another forty-five minutes.

Yield: 6 servings

Squash-Rice Luncheon

Baked Acorn Squash,	1 cup hot cooked white
Low-Fat Version (page	rice
143)	

Prepare the acorn squash according to the recipe. Spoon 1 of the rice in the center of two luncheon plates, arranging a well each mound of rice. Scoop out the cooked squash from the she. Place one-half of the squash in the well of rice on each plate.

Yield: 2 servings

Steamed White Rice

1 cup white rice   1 teaspoon salt
1½ cups water

Wash and drain rice. Place in the top of a double boiler. Cook until all the water is absorbed. Test for doneness by pressing a grain of rice between the fingers to make sure it is soft. For extra nourishment, rice may be cooked with skimmed milk instead of water.
Yield: 4 servings

Sauces, Dressings, Icings, and Frostings

Low-Fat Cottage Cheese Dressing

1 cup low-fat cottage cheese   2 tablespoons fresh lemon juice
½ cup buttermilk

Combine the ingredients. Blend until smooth.
Yield: 1½ cups

Mock Whipped Cream Topping

See page 128.

Pink Lady Topping

See page 129.

Rum-Flavored Mock Whipped Cream Topping

See page 128.

Low-Fat Tomato Sauce

1	twenty-ounce can tomatoes, drained	½	teaspoon allspice
½	teaspoon salt	2	tablespoons cornstarch
		2	tablespoons lemon juice

Simmer the tomatoes with the salt and allspice in a medium saucepan for about five minutes. Push through a sieve or a food mill. Blend the cornstarch with a little cold water in a small bowl. Add a cupful of juice from the strained tomatoes. Mix well. Combine the tomatoes and the cornstarch mixture in the medium saucepan. Cook until smoothly thickened. Stir in the lemon juice. Simmer for another five minutes, stirring occasionally.

Yield: 2½ cups

Low-Fat Yogurt Sauce

1	eight-ounce carton unflavored low-fat yogurt	2	tablespoons finely chopped parsley
2	tablespoons lemon juice		Dash of paprika
1	teaspoon salt		

Combine all the ingredients. Mix thoroughly. Serve the sauce immediately. Do not heat.

Yield: 1 cup

Lemon Icing

1	egg white	1	cup confectioners' sugar
1	teaspoon lemon juice		

Beat egg white until frothy. Sprinkle with lemon juice. Gradually beat in sugar until stiff enough to spread.

Yield: about ¾ cup

Mamma's Special Icing (Low-Fat Version)

See page 130, but substitute skimmed milk for the milk.

Suggested Daily Menus

1

Breakfast   1 glass pineapple and orange juice
strained oatmeal with skimmed milk and brown sugar
white bread with low-fat cream cheese and grape jelly
Sanka with skimmed milk

Lunch   Rice Carioca (ground beef and vegetables) (page 163)
2 slices white toast with 1 teaspoon margarine
Delectable Apricot Whip (page 157)
Tea

Dinner   Cream of Oyster Soup (page 135)
oysterette crackers
Baked Haddock (page 147)
canned stewed tomatoes
Steamed White Rice (page 164)
1 teaspoon margarine
strawberry Jello
Sanka with skimmed milk

2

Breakfast   ½ grapefruit
Cream of Wheat with skimmed milk and sugar
1 slice white toast with honey and 1 teaspoon margarine
coffee (if permitted) with skimmed milk

Lunch   Vegetable Beef Soup (page 137)
saltines, 1 teaspoon margarine
Pear and Cheese Salad (Low-Fat Version) (page 153)
Orange-Tapioca Pudding (page 159)
glass skimmed milk

Dinner   Turkey Casserole (page 143)
(rice and vegetables)
cranberry jelly

166

1 slice white bread with
1 teaspoon margarine
Hot Peach Dessert (page 158)
Tea

3

Breakfast   Banana broiled with honey
Puffed Rice with skimmed milk and sugar
Parker House roll with 1 teaspoon margarine
Sanka with skimmed milk

Lunch   Tomato Bisque (page 136)
Cod Fillets with Mushroom Sauce (page 147)
1 small baked potato with
1 teaspoon margarine
Baked Acorn Squash (Low-Fat Version) (page 143)
Grape Gelatin Special (page 157)

Dinner   Panbroiled Beef Patty (page 41)
on hamburger roll with 1 teaspoon margarine
Mixed Fruit Salad (Low-Fat Version) (page 151)
Tea (with sugar and lemon if desired)
low-fat lemon yogurt

4

Breakfast   stewed prunes
farina with skimmed milk and sugar
2 slices cinnamon toast (prepared without butter),
made of white bread
1 teaspoon margarine
coffee (if permitted) with skimmed milk

Lunch   Turkey Bone Soup (page 137)
Asparagus Salad (Low-Fat Version) (page 151)
1 soft roll
1 teaspoon margarine
Brown Betty (page 156)
1 glass skimmed milk

Dinner   Maple-Glazed Lamb Steak (page 141)
Party Green Peas (page 95)
Mashed Carrots (page 145)
1 small baked potato with
1 teaspoon margarine
Meringued Cherries (page 158)

Breakfast Baked Stuffed Pear (page 105)
cooked cornmeal with light brown sugar and skimmed milk
2 rusks
1 teaspoon margarine
coffee (if permitted) with skimmed milk

Lunch Carrot-Spinach Surprise (page 161)
sliced cold turkey
2 slices white toast
1 teaspoon margarine
low-fat yogurt, unflavored
1 cup tea with sugar

Dinner London Broil à la John (page 141)
1 small baked potato with 1 teaspoon margarine
Newport Spinach (page 145)
Marmalade Beets (page 145)
New England Apricot Pudding (page 159)
Sanka with skimmed milk

6

Breakfast 1 glass orange juice
Steamed White Rice (page 164)
with skimmed milk and brown sugar
1 egg scrambled in top of double boiler
1 slice white toast
1 teaspoon margarine
coffee (if permitted) with skimmed milk

Lunch Cream of Tomato Soup (page 35)
(made with skimmed milk)
Baked Oysters with Spinach (page 149)
1 slice white bread with
1 teaspoon margarine
tea
vanilla cornstarch pudding made with skimmed milk

Dinner Jelly-Glazed Roast Lamb (page 140)
Succotash (page 147)
canned peas and carrots
small boiled potatoes

1 teaspoon margarine
Apple Whisk (page 154)
tea (with sugar and lemon if desired)

7

Breakfast	stewed apricots Cream of Rice with skimmed milk and sugar 1 poached egg on 1 slice toast with 1 teaspoon margarine coffee (if permitted) with skimmed milk
Lunch	Macaroni and Tomato Luncheon (page 162) Individual Meat Loaf (page 140) 1 slice day-old white bread with teaspoon margarine Baked Stuffed Apple (page 156) 1 glass skimmed milk
Dinner	Cold Asparagus Soup (135) Plain Broiled Chicken (page 141) Green Beans and Mushrooms (page 144) mashed potatoes, prepared with 1 teaspoon margarine and skimmed milk Angel Food Cake (page 160) coffee (if permitted) with skimmed milk

Recipe Index

Recipe Index for the Bland Diet for Peptic Ulcer

177

Recipe Index for the Bland Low-Residue Diet

182

Recipe Index for the Bland Low-Fat Diet

190